SLEEPING YOUR WAY TO THE TOP

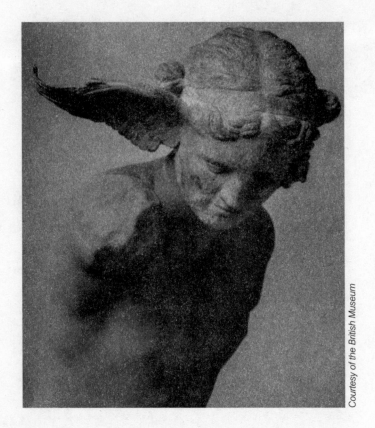

Hypnos (Somnus), god of sleep

The bronze winged head was found near Perugia, Italy, and was
acquired by the British Museum in 1866. The head is mounted
on a body that was copied from a statue with a similar head.

SLEEPING YOUR WAY TO THE TOP

HOW TO GET THE SLEEP YOU NEED TO SUCCEED

TERRY CRALLE, RN, and W. DAVID BROWN, PhD, with WILLIAM CANE

STERLING
New York

STERLING
New York

An Imprint of Sterling Publishing
1166 Avenue of the Americas
New York, NY 10036

ISBN 978-1-4549-1848-6

Distributed in Canada by Sterling Publishing Co., Inc.
c/o Canadian Manda Group, 664 Annette Street
Toronto, Ontario, Canada M6S 2C8
Distributed in the United Kingdom by GMC Distribution Services
Castle Place, 166 High Street, Lewes, East Sussex, England BN7 1XU
Distributed in Australia by Capricorn Link (Australia) Pty. Ltd.
P.O. Box 704, Windsor, NSW 2756, Australia

For information about custom editions, special sales, and premium and corporate purchases,
please contact Sterling Special Sales at 800-805-5489 or specialsales@sterlingpublishing.com.

Manufactured in the United States of America

2 4 6 8 10 9 7 5 3 1

www.sterlingpublishing.com

This book is dedicated with the greatest love to Richard Fitzgerald Cralle III—my son, my friend, my inspiration, my hero. Your kindness, strength, wit, and brilliance—and my love for you—are unparalleled. It is the honor of my life to be your mother.

—Terry

This book is dedicated to my many brilliant mentors: John Herman, Howard Roffwarg, Milt Erman, Phillip Becker, Andrew Jamieson, Michael Sateia, and Teofilo Lee-Chiong. Also to my children, David, Christopher, and Will, who had to sleep well to avoid my lectures.

—David

CONTENTS

PREFACE

During our combined thirty-five years of clinical practice in sleep medicine, we have been witness to something remarkable, so remarkable, in fact, that it prompted us to write this book to share it with a wider audience. As we treated patients over that time, we began to notice a definite pattern emerging: people who improved their sleep were more successful in their daily lives, including in school, in business, and in athletic and creative pursuits. We wrote this book to share our clinical experience about these findings and to let you know about the latest research in sleep science. This research generally confirms our clinical observations: getting sufficient sleep leads to an improved quality of life as well as increased productivity, creativity, and cognitive sharpness.

In order to illustrate various sleep principles, we have incorporated a few stories from our practice into the discussion. In each case, we changed names and identifying information, and in some cases we used composite characters drawn from our files. When we write in the first person, we always make clear who is speaking.

Part One is an overview of normal sleep and a look at the importance of sleep for optimal physical and cognitive performance. This part of the book debunks the notion that you can succeed by cutting back on sleep. Part Two covers sleep and athletic performance, and explains research that demonstrates how sleep can help improve mental and physical motor skills. Part Three covers sleep hygiene rules, as well as common sleep problems, including obstructive sleep apnea, insomnia, and restless legs syndrome. Along the way, we discuss clinically tested strategies for improving sleep, all of which are likely to make you more successful at whatever you do.

Here's to your good sleep!

—*Terry Cralle, RN*
—*William David Brown, PhD*

PART ONE

THE SEDUCTION
OF SLEEP

CHAPTER ONE

TRUMPING SLEEP

If you want to be a billionaire, sleep as little as possible.

—Donald Trump

Wealthy people sleep more than the nonwealthy.

—2013 Gallup Poll

Fact: most Americans sleep for failure. There are six reasons why they do so. They are unaware of the importance of sleep. They don't know the most effective methods of obtaining sleep. They suffer from common sleep disorders. They are inundated with blue light from electronic devices that degrades their production of the natural sleep hormone melatonin. They mistakenly believe that they can accomplish more if they sleep less. And last but not least, they live in a culture that devalues sleep.

This book makes a simple promise to you: it will inspire you to sleep for success. One of the chief methods that we'll use to help you consists of interpreting the latest sleep research for you in a way that can be immediately applied in your own life.

We are two sleep clinicians, and together we've worked with thousands of patients. They come to our clinics with sleep disorders, insomnia, sleep apnea,[1] and undiagnosed sleep difficulties. They sometimes are so sleepy that they fall asleep in our waiting rooms or while we're interviewing them. Some have experienced serious accidents due to poor sleep. Some have no idea why they have been referred to us; others want help, sometimes desperately, and we provide it—through sleep tests, sleep analysis, and sleep strategies that we and other professionals have developed over the years.

Sleep science has made exponential leaps in the past decade, but there are still questions that remain to be answered. Nevertheless, advances over the last few years have given us a far greater understanding of the importance of sleep. Even if you don't have major sleep problems, you'll soon discover that a better understanding of sleep will help you prioritize sleep and get the sleep you need to boost productivity and creativity, solve problems, and become more successful in all aspects of your life. To start, you must appreciate the importance of sleep.

All across America, people are laboring under a mistaken impression, one that's so ingrained in the modern psyche that it might as well be emblazoned across the twilight skies of our hometowns, writ large as if in huge skywriting letters:

THE LESS YOU SLEEP, THE MORE PRODUCTIVE YOU'LL BE

How this colossal myth has taken hold of the American Dream and nearly strangled the life out of it is the subject of this book.

With all the misinformation circulating in the media today, it's important that people with credentials debunk the fallacy that follows from this preposterous notion, namely:

SLEEP IS A WASTE OF TIME

In this book we provide concrete evidence that sleep is, instead, a fundamental need that can't be shortchanged without incurring serious negative consequences. Whether you're in the workplace, at home, or in school, if you wish to be a success, sleep needs to be your friend, not your foe.

Let's start with one cardinal principle that's easy to understand: *very few of us get as much sleep as we really need*. Without adequate sleep we risk not only our health but also the ability to feel, look, and do our best. We can't get to the top of anything if we're sleep deprived—and most of us don't even know that we *are*.

Many people believe they can function quite well on four to six hours of sleep per night. This is a myth. While the basal sleep need (the physiological amount of hours that are optimum for *you*) varies from person to person based on age, genetics, and perhaps other factors, it is known that adolescents, for example, need, on average, greater than nine hours of sleep[2] every night to perform optimally. A new study published in the journal *Sleep* indicates that adults need at least seven hours of sleep each night. For roughly ninety percent of the population, the optimal sleep requirement will vary from seven to nine and a half hours a night. It may also vary day by day, depending on various factors, including your state of health and whether you were sleep deprived during the previous few days, weeks, months, or even years.

Most of what we know about sleep has been discovered only in the past sixty years, and in that time compelling new research has come to light indicating that sleep may be one of the most important factors in the achievement of peak performance, optimum functioning, quality of life, and ultimate success. Scientists have only recently discovered the tremendous connections between sleep and high-performing individuals and organizations. Without a doubt, the implications of this research for your personal success are enormous. As sleep experts, we assure you that the correlation between the quality of sleep you get and the quality of life you lead cannot be overstated.

Largely ignored and devalued in American culture, sleep is slowly gaining recognition as the foundation of health and wellness that it really is. Indeed, it has recently received long-overdue credit as the third pillar in the health triad consisting of diet, exercise, and sleep. Despite the clear value of getting adequate sleep, some influential figures, from businesspeople to politicians to inventors, have attributed their success to short sleep or as little sleep as possible. Millionaire wannabes unwittingly and erroneously buy into this bravado, machismo, and air of superiority surrounding less sleep as a basis of success. This begs the question: Do we feel inadequate or destined to mediocrity because we need sleep or have an average sleep requirement?

> Don't think you will be doing less work because you sleep . . . That's a
> foolish notion . . . You will be able to accomplish more.
> —WINSTON CHURCHILL, Britain's prime minister,
> winner of the 1953 Nobel Prize in Literature

To best illustrate our point, we refer to a famous observation made by Donald Trump. Because of his success in the real estate world, he is often asked for advice by columnists, and his candor and controversial personality allow him to get plenty of attention in the media. Not surprisingly, he has weighed in on the subject of sleep and success. In a *Daily News* interview, he credits his success to sleeping only three to four hours each night in order to stay a step ahead of his competition. He says that he doesn't understand how sleep and success can coexist: "How does somebody that's sleeping twelve and fourteen hours a day compete with someone that's sleeping three or four?"

Well, Mr. Trump, here's our response. First of all, you may be a natural short sleeper.[3] According to sleep medicine experts, natural short sleepers are healthy people who sleep five hours or less per night. Short sleepers have a genetic variant that enables them to get by on very lit-

tle sleep. Studies have shown that individuals with this variant function well on very little sleep and seem especially adept at multitasking.
They're optimistic and outgoing and possess other similar traits that can
predispose them to success. Some studies, however, have suggested that
short sleepers may suffer from hypomania, a mild form of mania marked
by racing thoughts and few inhibitions. Hypomania is not necessarily a
positive condition. Although they may get very consolidated, restorative
sleep in the short time that they are asleep, people with hypomania can
experience a variety of negative symptoms (such as racing thoughts and
impulsiveness) along with their short sleep times. Despite these negatives, John Gartner, a psychiatrist at Johns Hopkins University Medical School, argues that hypomania generally gives people a competitive
edge.[4] So it's safe to assume that most of these individuals do have a
jump start on success, that is, they simply have more hours during the
day—to read, learn, think, research, go to school, you name it. The advantages in time alone are obvious, so it's logical that a lot of these folks do
shake out at the top. However, genetic short sleepers compose only about
three to five percent of the population, while long sleepers (who require
ten to twelve hours) comprise another five percent. *This means that forc-
ing yourself to be a short sleeper is not going to work for ninety-five percent of
the population.* In fact, attempting to deprive yourself of the amount of
sleep you genetically need is very likely to make you *less* successful. Note
that a short sleeper wannabe is far different from a true short sleeper
with the genetic variant.

Second, Mr. Trump, maybe you're exaggerating your claim about
not needing much sleep. You may simply be compensating by snoozing secretly during the day. Some people are more adept than others
at squeezing in a nap here and there. Weren't you even caught dozing
off in public at a recent tennis match between Venus and Serena Williams? Some folks who claim they need little shut-eye are actually getting more sleep than claimed and clearly don't function solely on three

to four hours. Others may require a steady supply of caffeine, sugar, or stimulants throughout the day, so that in spite of their claims of getting by on little sleep, they're not really "getting by"—they are compensating. Still others who claim not to need the typical amount of sleep may be experiencing performance decrements without even realizing it.

Third, Mr. Trump, with regard to success, we think you're looking at only one factor in the formula for success, namely the increased number of hours available to do things. We take the position that there is a great deal more to achieving success than extra hours during the day. While getting less sleep than needed does provide extra hours, it also results in sleep deprivation for people who have an average sleep requirement. So if we do the math correctly, we see that although fewer sleeping hours *will* add more waking hours, those waking hours are *diminished* in quality because of the physical and psychological consequences of sleep deprivation; as a result, success will be frustratingly unattainable. In fact, in the context of sleep deprivation, there is a decreasing return on the hours gained. If you have more time but are too tired or cognitively impaired to use it wisely, effectively, or efficiently, not only is nothing gained, but much is lost as sleep debt accrues.

So let's be clear. The majority of adults have a sleep requirement of around seven to nine hours. Meeting that requirement is more critical to success than having more hours to work. So we're here to tell you that Mr. Trump is dead wrong, and that boasting about needing very little sleep is doing more harm than good to the vast majority of people who want to be more successful and productive. Sleeplessness doesn't lead to success, nor does a normal sleep requirement preclude success. From a risk-benefit standpoint, *the benefits to your mental and physical health in trying to sleep less than needed do not outweigh the risks.*

Successful Sleep Rebels

Microsoft CEO Satya Nadella reportedly logs eight hours a night. Jessica Alba finds eight hours of sleep is important for reducing stress. Maya Angelou's bedtime was reported to be 10:00 p.m., with a wake time of 5:30 a.m. Heidi Klum reportedly requires ten hours per night, while Mariah Carey has been quoted as saying that fifteen hours of sleep is required for her to sing the way she wants to.

Facebook executive Sheryl Sandberg says that after years of skimping on sleep, she now aims for seven to eight hours of sleep nightly. It's reported that Beethoven turned in at 10:00 p.m. and awakened at 6:00 a.m. Tchaikovsky called it a night at midnight and woke up at 8:00 a.m. Basketball great LeBron James reportedly gets twelve hours of sleep per night, while tennis legend Roger Federer gets between eleven and twelve.

Instagram cofounder Kevin Systrom has been vocal about valuing sleep. In an interview with *People*, Matthew McConaughey finds that he needs eight and a half hours of sleep to perform at his best. Serena Williams told a UK reporter that she enjoys her sleep and turns in as early as 7:00 p.m. A true night owl, F. Scott Fitzgerald called 3:30 a.m. bedtime but slept until eleven the next morning. Charles Darwin slept eight to nine hours a night and napped daily from three to four in the afternoon.

B. F. Skinner hit the hay at 9:30 p.m. and slept until 6:30 a.m. Winston Churchill, John D. Rockefeller, Ronald Reagan, John F. Kennedy, and Napoleon also took naps in the afternoon to make up for their late nights.

Clearly success does *not* require cutting back on sleep time.

We know that today about 20 percent of Americans report that they get less than six hours of sleep on average, and the number of Americans that report that they get eight hours or more has decreased. While the exact, optimal number of sleep hours varies from person to person, the American Academy of Sleep Medicine is recommending that adults get at least seven hours of sleep each night. But if you listen to Donald Trump, you're likely to feel guilty about sleeping and you might try an ineffective strategy, such as sleeping only four or five hours. This would be a serious mistake for two reasons. First, *it's impossible to condition yourself to getting less sleep than you need*. Remember your sleep requirement is a biological necessity, not a test of willpower. And second—even more importantly—*success in life is dependent on the amount and quality of your sleep, so cutting back on the hours you spend snoozing is tantamount to setting yourself up for failure.*

This book is a collaboration between certified clinical sleep educator Terry Cralle, RN, and sleep psychologist William David Brown, PhD. It presents the information needed by motivated, driven, achievement-oriented, and ambitious people—anyone wishing to attain success and improved quality of life on any level. Based on compelling new research, this book's message is an urgent call to prioritize sleep for personal self-improvement, presented with applicable sleep strategies. If you hope to achieve success on any level, you must be unapologetic about your physiology, removing the stigma from your need for sleep, making sleep a new status symbol and priority.

Keep this intriguing fact in mind: successful people sleep *more* than the unsuccessful. A recent Gallup poll reveals that the wealthy sleep more than the poor.[5] But financial well-being is only *one* aspect of success. According to Tom Rath, a senior scientist and advisor to Gallup, and Jim Harter, PhD, Gallup's chief scientist for workplace management and well-being, success is also measured by advancement in the realms of career, social contacts, physical health, and community involvement.[6]

Throughout this book we will provide evidence that sleep contributes significantly to all these parameters of success, and more.

Secret Sleepiness

So if we're not able to willfully shorten our sleep needs, how is it that some successful people claim not to need sleep, or to need very little of it? What is their secret? One possibility is that they have lost their point of reference for feeling well rested. Dr. Tim Roehrs of Henry Ford Health System conducted research demonstrating that self-assessment of sleepiness is difficult and very often inaccurate. An objective sleep study called the multiple sleep latency test (MSLT) was conducted on research subjects who denied having any daytime sleepiness. Despite this, the results of the MSLTs revealed that 65 percent of the test subjects objectively demonstrated significant daytime sleepiness, while only 20 percent demonstrated normal results (meaning no daytime sleepiness). When the research subjects who were shown by the test to be sleepy increased their sleep time for one to two weeks, the repeated test results were normal, proving that those test subjects had indeed been sleepy, although they had not admitted to it and may not have recognized it.

CHAPTER TWO

PURE, UNADULTERATED SLEEP

The number of hours passed in sleep varies from six to twelve. The indolent, and those whose avocations or fortunes doom them to inert life, sleep many more hours than are necessary. But eight or nine hours would seem to be about the fair proportion, which every man ought to take, who values his health, or expects his intellects to be in a fit state to enjoy life.

—Dr. Edward Binns, *The Anatomy of Sleep* (1842)

In my practice as a sleep psychologist, I'm frequently amazed that people don't know what is normal or abnormal about sleep. I forget that most people don't spend most of their day studying sleep. It's important to have a basic understanding about what normal sleep is like. But first I'd like to share a little history with you.

When I was just starting to work, sleep studies were recorded on paper by ink pens, and you could actually hear when people went into REM sleep. You could tell something about the sleep stages just by listening to the pens on the paper. The sound of people going into REM was strik-ing: the pens stopped making noise when someone became paralyzed in REM stage sleep. When a patient moved in bed, ink would go flying off the paper. A typical nighttime study used about a thousand pages. In those days, we didn't have the ability to view results in expanded or compressed formats since we weren't recording with computers. I would unfurl the papers down the length of the hallway to see the entire night of sleep. And that brings me back to the subject of normal sleep.

If you watch someone sleep, they often look dead. If you ask about sleep, most people can't tell you much. "I got in bed and the next thing I knew, it was time to get up." The use of the electroencephalograph (EEG) changed all of our beliefs about normal sleep. An EEG records electrical currents in the brain through electrodes attached to the head. When we used the EEG, we no longer had to depend on our eyes or ask the subject. We had a way to actually watch the sleeping brain. When we started watching the brain during sleep, it became clear that the brain does not turn itself off during the night. In fact, at times the brain is more active than during wakefulness. As we continued to watch, we real-ized that all good sleepers follow the same path through the night.

A TYPICAL NIGHT

A good sleeper will usually fall to sleep fairly quickly. We don't consider it a problem until it takes well over thirty minutes on a regular basis to get to sleep. Once asleep, we descend very quickly through the first two stages to stage 3 sleep. This is a very deep sleep stage. It is difficult to awaken from, and if you do, you will be sluggish and disoriented. We even use the term *sleep drunkenness* to describe this feeling.

It is normal to awaken during the night. Most good sleepers awaken between five and eleven times each night. This doesn't mean they become fully alert, but they may open their eyes and change body positions, then

:kly return to sleep. The reason that we are unaware of this is that sleep has amnestic properties. That is, we forget what happens immediately before we fall asleep. If we awaken briefly, turn over, and go back to sleep, this event is wiped from memory and we feel as though we slept without waking throughout the night.

About ninety minutes after we fall asleep, the first REM period occurs. REM stands for rapid eye movement sleep and is so named because the eyes move rapidly. This is the stage in which dreams occur. The first REM period is usually quite short, three to five minutes. We then go back to stage 3 sleep. As the night progresses, we regularly enter REM sleep every ninety minutes. The amount of stage 3 sleep decreases and the amount of REM sleep increases. REM periods get longer as the night progresses, so that by morning a typical REM period may last thirty to forty-five minutes.

SLEEP STAGES

The night is filled with various sleep stages. The names of these stages have changed over time. Today, we use the following nomenclature.

STAGE 1 NREM SLEEP

NREM is non-rapid eye movement sleep, also known as Non-REM. This is the lightest and least refreshing sleep stage. In this stage you may be fantasizing about something or feeling pleasantly relaxed. If someone comes into your room, you would almost immediately awaken and say, "I just dozed off." If you spent the entire night in stage 1 sleep, you would not feel that you had slept well, or at all. We spend 5 to 10 percent of the night in this sleep stage.

STAGE 2 NREM SLEEP

This is a more solid sleep stage taking up about 50 percent of the night. If someone woke you from this stage, you would clearly feel that they woke you out of sleep. An EEG phenomenon called a K-complex is a marker of stage 2 sleep; it is an electrical discharge that is perfectly normal and occurs spontaneously. However, you can also cause a sleeper to produce a K-complex by making a loud, sharp noise such as clapping your hand. We think a K-complex is the brain trying to keep us asleep despite minor environmental noises or disturbances.

STAGE 3 NREM SLEEP

This is a deep sleep stage that occurs early in the night. It is sometimes called slow wave sleep (SWS) because the brain produces slower waves than at other periods of sleep. During this sleep stage, growth hormone is released. That means if you don't get stage 3 sleep, your body may not get growth hormone. This is obviously important for children; however, this stage is also important for adults. There may be an association between growth hormone, bone density, and muscle mass. There is an about 40 percent decline in slow wave sleep during the teenage years, and the amount of time spent in this sleep stage will continue to decline as we age. It is not uncommon to see normal sleepers after the age of forty get no stage 3 sleep at all. It normally composes 5 to 10 percent of total sleep time. It is increased when we are sleep deprived.

One way we tell the depth of a sleep stage is by the size and frequency of the EEG wave. Wakefulness is very low-amplitude fast activity. As we go to sleep, the frequency of the waves decreases and the amplitude increases. Stage 3 sleep is slow waves with high amplitude.

Another method is to see how loud a tone it takes to wake you out of the sleep stage. One study of children let them go to bed with earphones. Researchers sounded progressively louder tones to try to awaken the children. They stopped the study when they got to 123 decibels because they were worried about the children's ears. They were sleeping well. The tone was the equivalent of artillery fire.

> If sleep does not serve an absolutely vital function, it is the greatest
> mistake that evolution ever made.
>
> —ALLAN RECHTSCHAFFEN, PhD,
> pioneer sleep researcher at the University of Chicago

STAGE REM SLEEP

As mentioned, REM sleep is named for the rapid eye movements that occur during this stage. It is during REM that dreams occur. We are paralyzed in REM sleep. If you have ever dreamed of running away from someone, and you feel as if your legs are in molasses, you are responding to the atonia of this sleep stage. The body purposely turns our muscles off so that we can have these vivid hallucinations (dreams) without physically acting them out.

There is a disorder where people *can* move in REM sleep, and it is remarkably dangerous. I saw a patient who dreamed of diving and dove headfirst off of his bed. Another patient came in with his wife; he was very nice, but his wife had two black eyes. He would dream about being in combat and would start hitting his wife until she could manage to wake him.

Sleep researcher David Foulkes observed that dreams can also occur in NREM sleep. However, it seems that the "dreams" from NREM sleep are much less interesting. They're more like a thought—"I was sitting at my desk"—as opposed to the richness of the REM dream, in which there is often a story, characters, action, and bizarre occurrences.

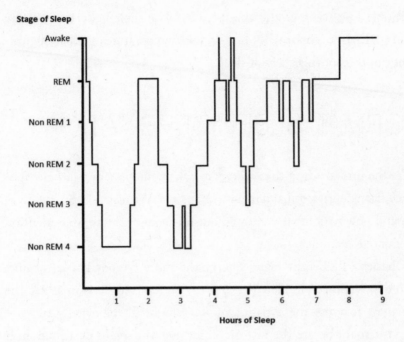

This sleep chart (hypnogram) illustrates a typical night of normal sleep.

The EEG waves of REM sleep are low amplitude and fairly random, making it seem like light sleep. But it takes a loud sound to wake you up out of REM sleep, so in this respect it also resembles deep sleep. If the sound has meaning, however, it doesn't have to be loud at all. For example, if someone whispers your name when you're in REM sleep, you'll likely awaken. It appears as if we're monitoring our environment during this sleep stage to see if there is something we need to wake up for.

We consider REM a "good" sleep stage because it is fragile; that is, many things can disrupt stage REM sleep. Both stage 3 sleep and REM sleep will rebound if suppressed. This means that if you had a night when someone woke you up out of REM every time you went into it, the next night you would have a great deal more REM sleep than normal. REM composes 20 to 25 percent of sleep time, and this percentage remains constant through a person's life cycle.

People lose some of the ability to regulate their body temperature during REM, so abnormally hot or cold temperatures in the environment can disrupt this stage of sleep.

NORMAL SLEEP DEPRIVATION

We're the first to admit that everyone will, at one time or another, experience sleep deprivation and incur a sleep debt. We discuss sleep deprivation and how to combat it throughout this volume. Here we'll mention one famous example.

Charles Lindbergh waged one of the more famous battles against sleep deprivation as he flew the *Spirit of St. Louis* to Paris in 1927. The first pilot to cross the Atlantic alone, Lindbergh reportedly did not sleep the night before the historic flight due to nervous anticipation. It is reported that he felt complete dread eighteen hours into the flight, realizing he still had an anticipated eighteen hours left to remain awake. Describing what today we call "microsleeps," Lindbergh later wrote about falling asleep with his eyes open. As his battle to stay awake continued, he skimmed waves with his plane, opened the plane's windows, scooped water onto his face, and resorted to holding his eyelids open with his fingers. He started hallucinating that ghosts were passing through the cockpit at around the twenty-four-hour mark of the flight. After thirty-three and a half hours of flying, and fifty-five hours of being awake, he landed in Paris and was quoted as saying that one of the greatest problems he experienced during the flight was staying awake.

Behind all too many disasters in the news are an array of mistakes blamed on sleep deprivation. We hear shocking stories about the lack of sleep among air traffic controllers, medical residents, bus drivers, and others, and realize that disasters like the *Exxon Valdez* oil spill, Three Mile Island nuclear meltdown, and Space Shuttle *Challenger* explosion were, at least in part, the result of sleep deprivation. It is in everyone's interest that the people who control transportation, energy, safety, education, health care, and government understand the critical importance of sleep. Clearly the recognition and reprioritization of sleep health is imperative to both individuals and society.

Short Sleep and Hypomania

Nikola Tesla, one of the world's foremost inventors, claimed to sleep just two to three hours per night. One of his biographers claimed that he stayed awake for eighty-four hours working on one invention.

But are short sleepers really more productive than the rest of us? Dr. Daniel J. Buysse of the University of Pittsburgh studied short sleepers in 2001. His research involved twelve confirmed short sleepers and twelve control subjects. A test titled Attitude for Life was administered to the study participants; it was actually a test for hypomania, which is a low-intensity mania characterized by fast talking, racing thoughts, and lowered inhibitions. *The short sleepers scored twice as high on the hypomania test as the control group.* One can't help but consider a bout of creative mania followed by long recovery sleeps and recuperative naps as an explanation for Tesla's eighty-four-hour work-a-thon.

Increase your sleep by as little as half an hour, or even fifteen minutes, if you can. Or get an extra hour of sleep every night for one week and see how immediate and drastic the benefits of extra sleep are.

The Two Factors of Sleep Control

Two physiological factors control sleep: one is homeostasis, the other circadian rhythms.

Homeostasis can be understood by considering that the longer you go without something, the stronger the drive to achieve it becomes. The best example of this is appetite. Appetite is a homeostatic drive. When you go a long time without eating, you get hungry. When you eat, the drive is decreased and you are satiated. A similar phenomenon occurs with sleep. *The longer you go without sleep, the greater the drive to achieve sleep becomes.* Well over one hundred years ago, it was demonstrated that if you deprived an animal of sleep, took some of its cerebrospinal fluid, and injected that fluid into a well-rested animal, the well-rested animal would fall asleep. The implication of this demonstration is that *something appears to build up in the bloodstream with sleep deprivation*.

We still don't know what the substance is, and the accumulation is probably more than a single thing. However, one attractive candidate is the chemical adenosine. Adenosine is the *A* in ATP, the energy molecule of the body. Adenosine makes people sleepy. Caffeine blocks adenosine receptors and makes you less sleepy. An area of the basal forebrain has been identified where extracellular levels of adenosine increase during the day and fall at night. While this is still controversial, the implication may be that sleep deprivation leads to the accumulation of some substance or substances (such as adenosine) that lead to sleepiness. Sleep somehow depletes these chemicals and results in alertness. This is likely a gross oversimplification of a complicated system, but for the purpose of demonstrating how a homeostatic drive could function, it is quite helpful.

The second factor that controls sleep is our *circadian rhythm*. Circadian means "about a day." The human clock runs at around 24.2 hours, not 24 hours, so it has to be reset every morning. There is a *circadian alerting rhythm* that directly counters the homeostatic sleep drive. As the sleep drive increases, the nervous system attenuates the drive by actively alerting the brain. The alerting tendency starts out fairly weak but gets progressively stronger into the evening hours. As bedtime approaches, these circadian alerting rhythms can be quite strong. In fact, "forbidden zones" are times during the twenty-four-hour day that sleep is almost impossible even in individuals that are sleep deprived. We tend to have forbidden zones in the late morning and early evening. This helps explain why it's often difficult to fall asleep when you go to bed at an earlier hour than your regular bedtime. It's usually easier to fall asleep when you stay up *later* than your normal bedtime.

At some point, the brain will turn the circadian alerting rhythms off. It may well be melatonin that does this. The brain produces melatonin when it gets dark and stops producing the hormone when it gets light. The human clock resides in a portion of the brain called the suprachiasmatic nucleus. If you drip melatonin on the suprachiasmatic nucleus, it will stop firing. This suggests that melatonin is, in fact, shutting down the circadian alerting rhythms. Once these alerting rhythms are switched off, the huge homeostatic sleep drive should now allow sleep to occur.

HOW YOU CAN HELP YOURSELF TO SLEEP

Although there are plenty of books and videos to help you diet and exercise, to date *sleep* health treatises for the general reader are virtually nonexistent. This absence of clinical evidence-based instruction to help people sleep better clearly reflects our culture's continuing lack of acknowledgment—and awareness—of the importance of sleep.

Now is the time for individual, cultural, corporate, and societal attitudes to catch up with the science of sleep. It's crucial for everyone to realize that the power of sleep has been proven, that negative effects of sleep deprivation cannot safely be ignored, and that quality sleep clearly outweighs the benefits of simply having more hours in the day. Obtaining an adequate amount of sleep through effective sleep management is the healthy, logical, and proven way to rise to the top.

Sleep Position and the Brain

Researchers have discovered that the brain has its very own detoxifying process, called the glymphatic system. Analogous to the lymphatic system, which flushes toxins from the body, the glymphatic system removes waste products from the brain while we sleep. New research from the University of Rochester in rodents has determined that the lateral, or side lying, sleep position promotes efficient waste removal.

CHAPTER THREE

SLEEP IS *NOT* A DIRTY WORD

Six for a man, seven for a woman, eight for a fool.

—Napoleon

The problem contemporary people face is that in a 24/7 society that values social media, late-night television, and burning the candle at both ends, well, let's face it, *sleep is a dirty word.* Not only has sleep been largely ignored and disregarded, but in American culture the need for sleep is seen as a weakness, even a character flaw. Perhaps a remnant of our Protestant work ethic, this negative attitude toward sleep pervades our culture as well as our psyches on both personal and professional levels. *In fact, a lack of sleep is one of the predominant and defining features of America's business culture.*

This negative view of sleep isn't new. The dark side of sleep is adeptly illustrated in *The Nightmare* by Henry Fuseli (1781), considered one of the classic depictions of sleep paralysis, with sleep portrayed as a frightening creature sitting on the chest of a sleeping woman (fig. 1). (Sleep paralysis is a temporary inability to move, experienced upon awakening or falling asleep.) Our everyday vernacular includes many negative references to sleep. We "wake up on the wrong side of the bed," put our sick and suffering animals "to sleep," and are advised to "sleep tight and don't let the bedbugs bite." "Sleeping with the fishes" implies death, or even murder. Warren Zevon sang "I'll Sleep When I'm Dead," and sleep has been referred to as a dress rehearsal for death.

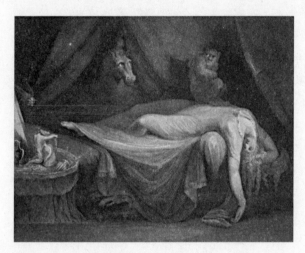

Figure 1. *Henry Fuseli's* The Nightmare *(1781)*

"Six for a man, seven for a woman, eight for a fool," said Napoleon. He obviously considered sleep a dirty word and viewed it as the ultimate limitation—both for himself and for his troops. Benjamin Franklin weighed in on the topic, if not a bit self-righteously, saying there would be plenty of time to sleep when he was dead. Franklin has no doubt been a source of frustration to every night owl with his infamous "Early to bed and early to rise makes a man healthy, wealthy, and wise." This statement reflects a curious double standard: *Why is being in bed by nine at night viewed favorably, while still being in bed at nine in the morning implies laziness?*

Sleep is the Rodney Dangerfield of medicine. It just gets no respect.

—JOHN WINKELMAN, medical director,

Sleep Health Center, Brigham and Women's Hospital

SLEEP—LAST BUT NOT LEAST

When people find out that we treat sleep problems, a common response is, "Oh, I have no need of your services. I can sleep anytime and anywhere without a problem." As soon as I hear this, I always smile to myself and think, *Well, it sounds like you have a little sleep problem right there, friend, and it may be precisely our services that you need.*

It also seems ludicrous that we condone smoking breaks at work, yet we find the biological need for sleep unmanageable. There are coffee breaks but not nap breaks. We employ people on twelve-hour shifts yet turn a blind eye to their safety as they drive home from work. It's unfortunate that we are pressured to improve our productivity by working more when our productivity would actually be improved with more sleep.

Why has sleep taken a backseat to diet and exercise? Ironically, research demonstrates that lack of sleep contributes to weight gain. Also, who wants to exercise when they're tired? Most people with sleep disorders and chronic sleep debt are not up at 5:00 a.m. to hit the gym before work. Rather, they're the ones who drag themselves out of bed in the morning feeling exhausted and consume caffeine and sugar to get through the day, only to come home and fall asleep in front of the television. In our practice, we find many patients come to the sleep lab so habituated to sleeping in their favorite recliner that they can no longer sleep in a bed.

It is imperative that we take the stigma out of our need for adequate, quality sleep. Too many people have lost their reference point for feeling well rested, and instead they muddle through the day, oblivious to the fact that sleep deprivation is the reason behind their problematic professional relationships, their struggle to focus on assignments, their moodiness and irritability, and their inability to lose weight and get to the gym.

SERIOUSLY SLEEPING

We push back waves of sleep as if they were a tsunami that would wash away all the great achievements within our grasp. But sleep is not an option—it is a biological *necessity*. It is not a sign of laziness or lack of willpower. It is a means to intelligence, strength, achievement, and success. Individually and as a society, we require, and gain from, adequate sleep. In the chapters ahead we will show that the more adequately we sleep, the more we accomplish and the better we are at whatever we do.

As a result of recent strides in sleep research, the role that sleep plays in health is finally gaining some recognition, albeit not nearly enough. Analogous to our approach to alcohol and cigarettes, behaviors we once tolerated will hopefully become unacceptable in the near future. Smoking is now prohibited in many public places, and we have come to understand the dangers of drunk driving. Yet while permitting a stumbling drunk to leave a bar and get in a car to drive home is a thing of the past, we don't think anything of allowing a worker to drive home on the brink of exhaustion after a twelve-hour shift. Is an inadvertent microsleep while driving drowsy any safer than driving drunk? The number of drowsy driving crashes rivals those related to alcohol, yet we still have not grasped the gravity of the situation. As long as there is a lack of awareness, the individual and societal consequences of sleep problems will persist.

The fact remains that adequate sleep is necessary to life. In this way it is similar to food. Even small reductions in the amount of sleep we get cause serious deleterious effects, and those few extra hours in the day that we acquire through reduced sleep can't begin to make up for the many negatives we suffer. We need to raise awareness and proactively manage this part of our lives in the same way we do diet, exercise, relationships, and careers.

Sleep is a criminal waste of time. A heritage from our cave days.

—THOMAS EDISON

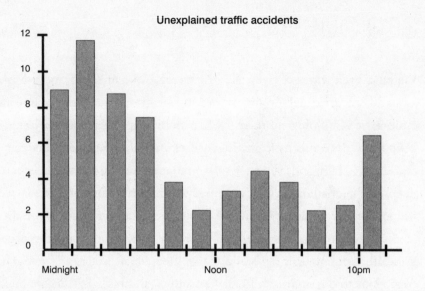

More unexplained accidents occur during periods when drivers can be expected to be sleepy.

Sleep is so integral to overall health and well-being that Dr. David Rye at Emory University School of Medicine encourages doctors to assess it at every medical appointment. His philosophy, with which we agree wholeheartedly, elevates sleep to a *vital-sign status*—precisely where it belongs. Unfortunately, our society's beliefs about sleep are categorically different from our approach to diet and exercise. And if we persist in missing the message about sleep's value, we're unlikely to practice sleep self-help in any meaningful way.

DIABETES AND SLEEP

Diabetes will soon be the number-one health problem facing the world, and obesity is already more prevalent than at any time in history. While the cause of type 2 diabetes is unclear, studies are also showing that *lack of sleep can contribute to the incidence of the disease*. A compelling case for the connection between diabetes and poor sleep is made in *Lights Out:*

Sleep, Sugar, and Survival (2001). In that treatise, T. S. Wiley and Bent Formby cite a multitude of studies indicating that lack of sleep contributes measurably to the incidence of diabetes. One of their conclusions is that loss of sleep destroys the endocrine balance that regulates weight gain.[1] These findings are in consonance with recent research revealing an improvement in insulin resistance after sleep is enhanced by treating obstructive sleep apnea.[2] Compelling new research also reveals an association between getting sufficient sleep and reduced rates of developing symptomatic diabetes.[3] With the rate of diabetes now considered an epidemic, it is clear that better sleep should play at least a contributory role in its treatment.

Sleep researcher Eve Van Cauter at the University of Chicago has examined the relationship among sleep, obesity, and diabetes. She found that sleep and metabolism are intimately connected. Most notably, sleep-deprived animals substantially increase the amount of food they consume. Sleepy humans have the same propensity to overeat. Many studies have demonstrated a correlation between total sleep time and BMI (body mass index): people getting the *least* amount of sleep tend to have the *highest* BMI. Sleep loss then seems to negatively influence the ability of the body to accurately perceive caloric need. Sleep-deprived people consume more calories than they need, and they gain weight as a result. These studies also tell us that sleep deprivation can be expected to make weight loss more difficult.

Two recently discovered hormones are known to regulate appetite and control body weight. Leptin is produced by adipose tissue (fat cells) and signals the brain that we don't need more food. It's an appetite suppressant. Ghrelin, on the other hand, is produced by the stomach and tells the brain that we do need more food. It's an appetite stimulant. Ideally, these two hormones should work in concert to create homeostasis. But even after only two days of partial sleep deprivation (four hours of sleep per night), leptin levels fall and ghrelin levels rise.[4] Basically, the sleep-deprived brain is being told that the person isn't eating enough, even though they may have consumed plenty of food. This leads to a desire for more food, particularly foods high in carbohydrates.

The ability of the body to remove excess glucose is called glucose tolerance. People with impaired glucose tolerance have trouble clearing sugar from their blood. This is a prediabetic condition. It turns out that sleep loss results in impaired glucose tolerance. A recent study examined healthy young men after six days of sleep curtailment (four hours of sleep). The ability of their bodies to clear glucose was 40 percent slower.[5] This study demonstrated a decrease in glucose tolerance and an increase in insulin resistance. In other words, in less than a week of sleep curtailment, healthy young men were put into a prediabetic state.

THE AMERICAN VIEW OF SUCCESS

For some reason Americans, especially those in the business world, blindly buy into the misconception that sleeplessness equates to success. Dr. Charles Czeisler, Baldino Professor of Sleep Medicine at Harvard Medical School, coined the term *sleepless machismo* to describe this attitude. He and other sleep experts are rightly frustrated by the double standard that pervades the corporate world: businesses have policies and assistance for workplace drinking, drugs, smoking, sexual harassment, bullying, maternity leave, and sick leave, *yet where is the comparable acknowledgment of sleep health?*

> I think sleeping was my problem in school. If school had started at four in the afternoon, I'd be a college graduate today.
>
> —GEORGE FOREMAN,
> two-time world heavyweight champion boxer

It is a fact that the very part of the brain that provides insight into our own state of mind shuts down when we're sleepy. Sleep-deprived (cognitively and physically impaired) people will run a country, fly a plane, take a test, participate in a debate, drive a car, remove a gallbladder, enact laws, operate machinery, and make important decisions under the influence of sleepiness—without realizing their level of impairment.

Prior to 1760, when new manufacturing processes ushered in the era of mass production, people slept more than we do today. With the advent of the Industrial Revolution, sleep time began to dwindle. The modern Prometheus, Thomas Edison, brought daylight indoors and made it affordable for everyone. Because workers could toil late into the night, their appreciation of the value of sleep became diluted. Such attitudes are now firmly entrenched as part of the American ethos. The title of Oliver Stone's film *Wall Street: Money Never Sleeps* (2010) gives voice to this misguided attitude.

By now, we trust you see eye to eye with us about the value of sleep. With that as our starting point, we're ready to pull out all the stops to help you become a winning sleeper. In the coming chapters, you'll learn how to get the sleep you need for increased productivity in every area of your life.

CHAPTER FOUR

NOT NOW, I'M TIRED

Drowsiness or sleep deprivation . . . is beginning to outstrip alcohol as a cause of accidents in transportation, particularly on the highway.

—Dr. William Dement, legendary sleep researcher

One afternoon I was surprised to notice a man who looked like Patrick Swayze sitting in the waiting room of our clinic. He was wearing a shirt and tie and appeared to be exhausted. Mr. L. explained that he hoped that I could give him some help with his sleep problems. He was forty-seven and complained about being exhausted. The problem had been getting worse over the last few years.

"What's your schedule like?" I asked.

"Up early for meetings, Terry. That, plus the day ends around ten. But I'm not sure I have a sleep problem. I can fall asleep anytime, anywhere."

"When you say you're exhausted, what does that mean? Is it low energy, malaise, lack of motivation, or is it sleepy?"

"I guess it's all of the above," he said. "I do my job well but meetings are murder. I load up on the coffee before one of those; they're sooo boring."

"How much sleep are you getting at night?"

"I go to bed at midnight and I'm asleep before my head hits the pillow. I get up at six. I've never needed much sleep."

"You don't think you need more sleep?"

"No! In fact, I always catch up on weekends by sleeping late, and I feel even worse when I do that. I've adapted to little sleep and I accomplish more when I get going early."

This is a typical conversation with patients. Mr. L. feels that he sleeps well because he falls asleep instantly and does not wake up during the night. He finds it difficult to awaken in the morning, but after his first two cups of coffee, he's "good to go." Even with several more cups of coffee during the day, he may nod off briefly, but only when "I'm completely bored. But who doesn't? If I'm active, I'm fine."

Mr. L. is clearly suffering from chronic partial sleep deprivation.[1] Even though he sleeps every night, he's getting less sleep than his body needs. Broadly defined, sleep deprivation is a condition caused by not getting enough sleep.[2] Insufficient or inadequate sleep can be the result of either reduced sleep time or poor sleep quality. Although people can grow accustomed to a sleep-deprived schedule, they cannot adapt to getting less sleep than needed. It is a biological impossibility. Sleep deprivation occurs when there's insufficient sleep to support an individual's health, alertness, performance, and overall functioning.

Sleep deprivation can lead to a condition known as local sleep. A relatively new area of investigation, local sleep is a disorder in which a specific *region* of the brain sleeps. It's now known that small portions of the brain can fall asleep while the rest of the brain remains awake. This is different from a microsleep, during which the entire brain of the organism is cut off from the environment. In local sleep, people can be going about their business but part of the brain may fall asleep. We really don't know the full consequences, but intriguing ideas are that during local sleep we might experience a loss of our train of thought, a slip of the tongue, brain farts, or senior moments.

I first had to convince Mr. L. that he was sleep deprived. Since he had always slept about six hours a night, he mistakenly believed that he had successfully adapted to this amount of sleep. Like most sleep-deprived people, he was unaware of his cognitive impairment. He was covering up his sleepiness by scheduling boring activities in the morning, consuming high levels of caffeine, and staying more active in the afternoon when his sleepiness was most pronounced. I informed him that a boring meeting, a warm room, or lunch does not make us sleepy. What these sedentary activities do is unmask latent sleepiness.

Reducing sleep deprivation will invariably improve your productivity at work. The first thing I mentioned was that studies with US Marines suggest that reducing sleep deprivation can result in improved work per-formance.[3] Mr. L. was impressed to learn that the studies had found that loss of sleep results in degraded job performance, and correcting sleep deprivation can result in improved work productivity.

"Remember," I began, "your wake-to-sleep ratio needs to be two to one. Adequate sleep—typically seven to nine hours of it—is required for our bodies and minds to function optimally, and a sufficient amount of sleep is mandatory for peak functioning. This is not just one or two nights of catching up. It needs to be consistent. That is, get an adequate amount of sleep every night, or at least most nights. Trying to change your body's need for sleep is futile, if not downright dangerous."

As we will soon see, sleep loss is cumulative. That is, every hour of sleep lost will begin to accumulate a sleep debt. And even a fairly modest sleep debt takes a long time to pay back.

"The first idea I want you to try," I told Mr. L., "is to avoid incurring sleep debt by keeping a consistent and adequate sleep schedule. But if you do lose sleep, try to make up for the loss as soon as possible. Also, you can practice sleep banking if you anticipate sleep loss. For example, if you have a hectic travel and meeting schedule approaching, you can extend your sleep time or take naps in anticipation of the unavoidable sleep loss."

Most sleep-deprived people don't feel sleepy and are unaware that they are operating at suboptimal physical and cognitive levels.

MAKE UP SLEEP LOSS ASAP

It's best to make up sleep loss as soon as possible in order to lessen the deleterious effects. I once heard William Dement, the father of sleep medicine, describe sleep debt as starting each morning with an empty backpack. Every hour that you're awake, you put one brick into the pack. By the end of the day, you've gathered sixteen bricks. For every hour that you sleep, two bricks are removed from the backpack. If you sleep eight hours, all sixteen bricks are removed and you start the day fresh. However, if you sleep only six hours, then only twelve bricks are removed and you start the day with four bricks in the backpack. If you continue to get only six hours sleep, you'll accumulate eighteen bricks per day but get rid of only twelve each night. You can see what a burden you begin each day with when you fail to get sufficient sleep.

What Is a Microsleep?

A microsleep is a brief episode of sleep that lasts for a fraction of a second to half a minute. You can see people experiencing a microsleep on the subway where their head will nod, and then they will wake up and sit up straight, only for the process to repeat. Other examples of a microsleep can occur when people lose their train of thought or have a blank stare. During a microsleep, a person fails to respond to the environment. It is one of the most dangerous consequences of sleep deprivation.

During a microsleep, the brain automatically shuts down, falling into a brief sleep state, usually followed by a period of disorientation. The person experiencing a microsleep falls asleep regardless of the activity they are engaged in. Microsleeps are similar to blackouts, and a person experiencing them is not consciously aware that they are occurring. The propensity for microsleeps increases as sleep debt accumulates. People often have their eyes open during a microsleep.

You have undoubtedly seen people in a microsleep. You are talking to them, their eyes are open, but you know no one is home. They have spaced out or tuned out. While a microsleep may last just a few seconds, during that time, the person is completely cut off from the world. In *The Promise of Sleep* (2000), William Dement describes a study in which a male volunteer was partially sleep deprived. He was then put on a table with his eyelids taped open. There was a strobe light just inches from his face. He held a button in his hand. His brainwaves were being monitored. The task was simple: when the strobe flashed, he would push the button. He started out getting 100 percent of the flashes correctly, but soon he began missing flashes. Keep in mind that his eyes were taped open. When he was asked why he did not push the button, he responded that it was because the light did not flash. For every miss, the EEG showed that his brain was asleep at the moment of the flash even for just a few seconds. This shows something remarkable. We feel as if we drift to sleep slowly. In reality, the instant the brain is asleep, it is cut off from the world, and it happens quickly. It feels like drifting because we have just a few seconds of sleep here and there before our brain is consistently asleep. This is important because if you experience a microsleep, you are oblivious to the outside world. The head bobbing and chin hitting the chest are not the first signs of sleep; rather, they are well into the sleep process.

SYMPTOMS OF SLEEP DEPRIVATION

The primary effect of sleep deprivation is excessive daytime sleepiness. A sleep-deprived person like Mr. L. is likely to fall asleep when forced to sit still in a quiet or monotonous situation, such as during a meeting or class. Note this distinction: a sleep-deprived person will fall asleep in a monotonous or boring situation, whereas a well-rested person will merely be bored. There are some subtle and not-so-subtle signs of sleep deprivation, including:

- Yawning, heavy eyelids, eye rubbing, head nodding, frequent blinking, eye closure, and involuntary microsleeps.
- Falling asleep in less than five minutes at bedtime.
- Dependency on an alarm clock and the snooze button.
- Requiring high levels of caffeine or other stimulants throughout the day.
- Eating candy and high-sugar snacks for energy.
- Language problems, slurred or monotonous speech, stuttering, needless repetition, and being at a loss for words.
- Being quieter and more withdrawn than usual.
- Vision blurriness, difficulty focusing, eyelid twitching.
- Impaired immune function; frequent colds and illnesses.
- Increased sensitivity to pain; feelings of vague discomfort.
- Problems with short-term memory and recall.
- Inability to focus, concentrate, or pay attention.
- Clumsiness, balance problems, lack of coordination.
- Reduced sex drive.
- Lack of judgment or insight.
- Feeling stressed.
- Falling asleep at inappropriate times.
- Irritability, mood swings, a short temper, depression, irrational behavior, paranoia, aggression, agitation, pessimism.
- Difficulty finishing tasks.
- Feeling drowsy while driving.
- Hyperactivity, feeling giddy, or acting intoxicated.

- Loss of situational awareness; reduced awareness of the environment.
- Regularly feeling exhausted by midafternoon.
- Shortened attention span.
- Impaired decision making.
- Mental stalling, that is, fixating on one thought.
- Errors of omission: making a mistake by forgetting to do something.
- Errors of commission: making a mistake by doing something but choosing the wrong option.
- Reduced work efficiency.
- Increased risk-taking behavior.

The Cumulative Nature of Sleep Loss

A study conducted by Thomas Alvin Wehr in the early '90s demonstrated both the cumulative nature of sleep loss and the time it may take to catch up. In this study, young men who averaged about seven and a half hours of sleep per night were required to stay in bed in a dark room for fourteen hours per day, every day for a month. The experiment was actually attempting to examine sleep patterns during the preindustrial winter months, a time when people's sleep and wake patterns were dictated more by the light-dark cycle. What was observed was that almost immediately, the young men began sleeping about twelve to thirteen hours per day. The second finding was that it took approximately three weeks before their total sleep time reached a plateau at about 8.25 hours. The immediate increase in sleep time suggested that even sleeping 7.5 hours each night can lead to sleep deprivation. It took three weeks to make up for this chronic though modest sleep deprivation. Chronic sleep deprivation means loss of sleep, sometimes without the person being aware of it, that has continued for a long time. Acute sleep deprivation, on the other hand, means loss of sleep for one or two nights. Trying to "catch up" over a weekend will help to some degree with chronic sleep deprivation, but it actually takes much longer to thoroughly eliminate such long-term debt.

GIVE YOURSELF MORE THAN ONE RECOVERY NIGHT

After two weeks of extending his sleep time, Mr. L. was noticing improvement in his exhaustion. He was still falling asleep quickly, but he could now read before bedtime. He required an alarm to wake up, but he no longer used the snooze button.

"I'm actually feeling more rested in the morning," he said. "I seemed to have forgotten what it was like to get up and feel good."

One of the most effective ways to improve your mental and physical condition is to allow sufficient recovery sleep. We're all under the illusion that we can catch up on our sleep over a weekend. Extending sleep for a couple of days does indeed help us feel better, but it hardly makes up for months or years of sleep loss. A key finding of another recent study was that a short rest pause or a night of recovery for chronically sleep-deprived people can be helpful, but it fails to return productivity to the level of people without sleep loss.[4] If sleep loss is acute (as opposed to chronic), researchers concluded that two nights of good sleep were sufficient to make up for this short-term sleep debt.

Chronic partial sleep deprivation can cause changes in the brain's neurotransmitter receptors. It takes a while to make these changes, and it will take a while to reverse the process. Common sense as well as research tells us that chronic sleep deprivation is worse than acute deprivation. For example, research by David Cohen and colleagues showed that if you're sleep deprived for a week or more (chronic deprivation) and then you get extra sleep for one day, followed by insufficient sleep again at the start of the new week, your impairment level is much worse than someone who had plenty of sleep in the weeks prior to the deprivation.

The point is that although you can make up for sleep loss, it takes longer than most people realize.[5] People who think they can compensate for chronic sleep loss with a single night or two of extra sleep are fooling themselves.[6]

I told Mr. L. that I was proud of his ability to extend his sleep time by two hours each night. He was going to bed an hour earlier and sleeping an hour later.

"You should continue to see improvement over the next several weeks, as long as you keep with the longer sleep schedule. A full recovery of chronic sleep deprivation takes time."

"Once I get this extra sleep, will I sell more beds?" he asked me.

I smiled. "I can't guarantee that," I said. "After all, I don't know how badly your clients need the beds. But if you mean will you be more effective at selling, then the answer is yes. In other words, if the client is ready to make a purchase and all he needs is someone to present the information in a calm and thorough manner, you'll certainly be in a better position to do that if you're fully recovered from your sleep debt."

Mr. L. became quite interested in his sleep as a result of the modest improvement he made in just two weeks. To keep better records of his sleep, I suggested that he track it with a sleep diary, app, or wearable device that monitors sleep. I also encouraged him to record how many sales he made, how difficult or easy it was to make them, and how rested or sleep deprived he felt each day.

He took my suggestion about a wearable device, and three and a half months later I received a letter from him thanking me for the advice I had given him. Using the tracking device had changed the way he managed his sleep as well as his work and leisure time. Although this is only anecdotal evidence, it is squarely in line with what other clients, and the research, clearly reveal. When you make up for sleep deprivation, you operate at your peak performance level. Your job will seem easier and become more fun. And you can expect to do it better.

Isn't it nice to know that you can give yourself a significant competitive advantage by getting some good sleep? Here's another way to look at it. When you go to bed, you don't have to worry that you're shirking your job responsibilities. No, just the opposite. By giving yourself time to recover from sleep deprivation, and by getting the restful sleep you need, you're actually working at improving your job productivity. You might even smile to yourself, since in this case "working" really means sleeping—and feeling good about it, too. "We love to work at nothing all day," said Bachman-Turner Overdrive, putting into words something rather profound that we can all take to heart. Often doing nothing (by which, of course, we mean *sleeping*) is actually the best thing you can do for your career.

RECOVERY

The recovery of sleep deprivation involves two distinct phases of rebound. On the first recovery night, participants show an increase in the percentage of slow wave sleep time while REM remains at normal levels. During subsequent nights, REM sleep percentage increases significantly over baseline levels, while slow wave sleep remains at normal levels. The makeup of slow wave sleep before REM during rebound sleep has been observed in many studies.

These findings suggest that there may be two distinct regulatory processes governing sleep—one that functions in the short term and one that is impacted by more cumulative sleep patterns across weeks and even months. The cause for concern is the fact that people who endure chronic sleep loss—people sleeping less than they need to over many weeks or months—may believe that they have fully recovered, but their performance continues to suffer from the long-term effects of too little rest.

We are living in the middle of history's greatest experiment in sleep deprivation and we are all part of that experiment . . . Sleep deprivation doesn't have any good side effects.

—DR. ROBERT STICKGOLD, *Harvard Magazine* (2005)

THE COST OF INSUFFICIENT SLEEP

A plethora of studies show the many negative effects that insufficient sleep has on our physical and mental functioning. We now know that sleep time is correlated with body mass index (BMI). People who sleep the least tend to have a higher BMI. Decreased sleep time is also associated with insulin resistance and poor glucose tolerance, increasing the risk of developing type 2 diabetes. Sleep-deprived people are much more likely to be involved in automobile accidents and work-related accidents. Insufficient sleep impairs attention, concentration, and memory. It predisposes people to depression and anxiety. Sleep deprivation clearly impairs performance on a number of cognitive and motor tasks such as reaction times.[7] Both short and long sleep times are associated with all-cause mortality. This means that deaths from all causes increase with sleep loss as well as with excess sleep.

Staying awake for nineteen hours produces performance deficits comparable to having a blood alcohol content (BAC) level of .05 percent; being awake for twenty-four hours, a BAC of .10 percent. The legal limit is .08 percent. Nationwide, for commercial drivers, a BAC of .04 percent can result in a DUI conviction. For those under twenty-one, there is a zero-tolerance limit—any amount of alcohol is grounds for a DUI arrest. It has been estimated that as many as 30 percent of our workforce is chronically sleep deprived. Safety officers for large companies would never let 30 percent of employees come to work intoxicated. Yet they may be letting employees come to work with an equivalent level of impairment caused by sleep loss without saying a word.[8]

You Don't Know What You're Missing

Sleep-deprived people do not realize their impairments. They lack insight into how sleepy they are and how it's affecting them.

Even relatively moderate sleep restriction can seriously impair waking neurobehavioral functions in healthy adults. *The important point is that feeling tired can feel dangerously normal after a short time.* Sleepiness ratings suggest that subjects are largely unaware of these increasing cognitive deficits, which may explain why the impact of chronic sleep restriction on waking cognitive functions is often assumed to be benign.

Many people are under the mistaken impression that they're capable of adjusting to less sleep, and they attempt to counteract the effects through caffeine, sugar, and other means. While caffeine may help counter the effects of sleepiness, it does not compensate for the other benefits that sleep confers, such as memory consolidation and emotional stability. Any sense of adaptation or adjustment is a falsehood, and this lack of self-awareness or skewed thinking can be directly attributed to sleep loss itself. As we have emphatically stated, sleep loss impairs our insight, judgment, and decision-making capabilities—the fundamental aspects of reasoning required to make sound decisions about everything, including our sleep. So we really have not adjusted to less sleep; our state of sleep deprivation fools us into thinking we have. Our subjective assessment of performance is inaccurate and completely unreliable, and physical and cognitive decline ensue.

Research clearly demonstrates the inability to adapt to sleep deprivation. If you aren't one of the few genetically natural short sleepers, then you have to be realistic about your need for sleep to maintain your health and functioning.

The best way to summarize this important research on sleep deprivation is to put it like this: *you don't know what you're missing.* No matter how intelligent you may be, you will not be able to perceive the nature and severity of the cognitive and performance impairment that you're experiencing. Even reading this book won't enable you to recognize how mentally impaired you are due to sleep loss.

HOW YOU CAN MAKE UP SHORT-TERM SLEEP DEBT

Dr. Lawrence J. Epstein at Harvard Medical School is an expert on how to compensate for sleep debt. I shared some of his research with Mr. L. The difference between short-term and long-term sleep debt is that short-term debt consists, for example, of missing about ten hours of sleep over the course of a week. Long-term debt would involve doing this regularly for a period of weeks or months.

Dr. Epstein recommends the following strategy to make up for short-term sleep loss. First, give yourself extra time to sleep on weekends. For example, you could add three or four hours of extra sleep on Saturday and Sunday. Although some researchers caution that sleeping past your usual wake-up time might throw you off your sleep schedule, it's more important that you quickly make up the lost sleep, and a good opportunity to do that is on the weekend. Since you're not doing it every weekend, it's unlikely to disrupt your sleep schedule and may, in fact, enable you to get back on track with that early-morning awakening time *without the alarm clock*. In addition to extra weekend sleep, you should also add an extra hour or two during each night of the next week. In this way you'll come out fully rested and ready to compete on the highest level, whatever your profession. Naturally this will only work if you change your sleep habits going forward and sleep appropriately.

Sleep Inertia

Sleep inertia is that groggy feeling you experience upon awakening. It can vary in length and severity depending on a number of factors. Basically, when the brain wakes, it does not come fully online immediately. Some portions of the brain return to alertness rather slowly. For the first five minutes after waking, people perform on cognitive tests about five standard deviations below the norm. This means that we're not processing information very effectively when we first awaken. So be careful what you say if the phone awakens you during sound sleep . . . you may regret it later.

HOW YOU CAN MAKE UP LONG-TERM SLEEP DEBT

For those who are chronically sleep deprived—including most Americans who get less than the optimal hours of sleep each night and who have been depriving themselves of sleep for months—there is another, more drastic strategy that Dr. Epstein recommends to make up this more significant sleep debt. The good news is that you're guaranteed to enjoy this method! You begin by scheduling a vacation. Ensure that you don't have to rise and shine or do any work during this interlude. Then sleep every day until you feel fully rested.

Most important of all, do not use an alarm clock to wake up during this vacation. Your goal is to make up the sleep debt and bring yourself to a point where you naturally awaken every day around dawn. In this way you will have readjusted your circadian clock to be on a natural sleep cycle.

Granted, not everyone has the luxury of taking a vacation for the purpose of getting back on track with their sleep schedule. However, for those who can take a few days off to try this technique, it is a proven way to fight back against the sleep deprivation that plagues modern humanity. You will boost your alertness and enjoy significant advantages over your competitors by recharging yourself in this manner.

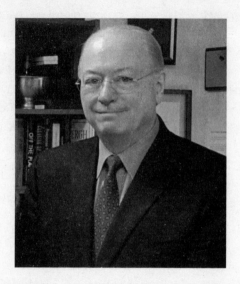

Dr. David F. Dinges, Perelman School of Medicine at the University of Pennsylvania, a major American sleep researcher, has illuminated the impact of sleep debt on cognitive function.

BOOSTING BRAIN FUNCTION

Dr. David F. Dinges is the director of the Unit for Experimental Psychiatry and chief of the Division of Sleep and Chronobiology at the Perelman School of Medicine at the University of Pennsylvania. He and his colleagues have discovered that even a few nights of sleep deprivation result in reduced brain activation in multiple regions, "including bilateral intraparietal sulcus, bilateral insula, right prefrontal cortex, medial frontal cortex, and right parahippocampal gyrus."[9] If this isn't enough to make you sit up and take notice of the harm of missing sleep, well—I don't know what is!

These brain regions control critical thinking and behavioral functions, including perceptual-motor coordination, directing eye movements, and reaching (bilateral intraparietal sulcus); consciousness, emotion, physical homeostasis, perception, motor control, self-awareness, and cognitive functioning (bilateral insula); personality, planning complex behavior, decision making, and social behavior (right and medial prefrontal cortex); and working memory, short-term memory, memory for spatial location, and the ability to detect sarcasm (right parahippocampal gyrus). Perhaps a simpler way of summarizing these findings might be to say that *sleep deprivation significantly reduces brain functioning*.

Dr. Dinges and his team also found that chronically sleep-deprived people mistakenly *thought* they were performing well when objectively they were as impaired as a person with one to two nights of total sleep deprivation.[10] The takeaway message is clear: you can enjoy a competitive advantage over others by ensuring that you're getting sufficient sleep on a regular basis. Doing so will put you ahead of your sleep-deprived competitors, improve your mood, and boost your brain functioning significantly above the level of many of the people around you.

Insufficient Sleep?
Here's How to Make It Up

If you need an alarm clock to wake up, have difficulty getting out of bed in the morning, feel tired during the day, and fall asleep the minute your head hits the pillow at night, you're probably not getting the amount of sleep you need.

To accurately assess your individual sleep requirement, don't set the alarm on the weekend. According to Dr. Robert Stickgold, if you don't set the alarm and you sleep more than you normally would during the week, you're liable to be getting an insufficient amount of sleep.

Give yourself more than two nights of extra sleep to make up for significant sleep debt. Your brain will function better and you'll be more capable of working and interacting with other people.

Making up significant sleep debt generally takes more than two nights. Getting that extra sleep has been shown to boost numerous

thinking and motor skills, including planning ability, the ability
to detect sarcasm, and your ability to remember where things
are. Although you may not feel that you need it, because we're
rarely able to accurately sense our own sleep deprivation, getting
sufficient makeup sleep will have measurable benefits for your
mind and body, increasing mental sharpness and physical reaction
time, among other important parameters of peak functioning.

CHAPTER FIVE

SLEEP AND GROW RICH

In both writing and sleeping, we learn to be physically still at the
same time we are encouraging our minds to unlock from the
humdrum rational thinking of our daytime lives.
—**Stephen King, *On Writing* (2000)**

A new patient came to see me because she was distraught over one of
her dreams.

"I dreamed last night that my mother died."

"Hmm," I said. I am a psychologist, after all.

"The dream worries me because my dreams tend to come true. I'm
certain that my mother is going to die soon."

"Has you mother been ill?"

"Yes, she's been struggling with cancer for more than a year. We've all
been worried sick about her."

This is a remarkably common conversation with people who have a
firm belief that their dreams are heralding a death or catastrophe. And
it's not a new phenomenon. We have evidence of dream interpretation
from clay tablets created in 4000 BC. Dreams have always held a special

place in our psyche. They were often believed to be messages from the gods or visions of the future. The study of dreams contributed to the emergence of the field of sleep medicine.

With the discovery of REM sleep, the physiological substrate of dreaming, our ability to study dreams improved exponentially. While there is still debate over the meaning (if any) of dreams, they continue to fascinate and sometimes terrify us. At a minimum, the totally different physiological state that occurs during sleep, particularly REM stage sleep, allows the brain to process information in a manner that may not be possible during the awake state.

SLEEP FOR SUCCESS

When faced with a difficult situation, you've undoubtedly heard the advice to "sleep on it." Where did that expression originate? And why is there a connection between sleep and problem solving?

The most obvious reason to sleep on a problem is to allow more thought time before making a decision. This so-called incubation period is critical to problem solving.[1] More thought time allows more options to be considered. But the advice to sleep on it goes beyond buying more time to mull over a problem. Might sleep *itself*, and not just the extra thought time, in some way add to and enhance the problem-solving and decision-making process? Current research suggests that the answer to this question is a resounding yes. It is now known, for example, that sleep itself functions to restructure problems, allowing new insights to be reached.

Until the mid-1950s, scientists generally assumed that the brain shut down during sleep. This erroneous idea most likely originated from the observation of sleeping people. Take our word for it, watching a person sleep is *not* fascinating—and we've watched hundreds of people sleeping in our sleep labs. If they aren't snoring, they often appear to be dead.

But in actuality the brain is exceedingly active during sleep—at times, even more so than during wakefulness. There appear to be unique associations and connections made during sleep which are not possible during the day. We now know that the brain is chemically very different during its sleeping and waking states. During sleep, there is a chemical shift in the predominate neurotransmitters that are communicating throughout the brain, including norepinephrine, serotonin, and GABA (an inhibitory neurotransmitter). This chemical change causes regions of the brain that are typically very active during wakefulness to be completely quiescent during sleep. The brain's use of oxygen and energy also changes during sleep—at times exceeding its energy consumption during wakefulness. These changes literally reroute our thought processes during sleep, causing a profound shift in mental calculations and, most importantly, an extraordinary ability to perceive problems in a slightly different manner. *This sleep-induced shift in perspective allows us to make connections that were not obvious when we were awake.* As such, sleep provides us with a way to examine and think about things in a manner that isn't possible for the awake brain. It is entirely possible, then, that one function of sleep may be to restructure problems and allow for new insight. Dreaming may be the brain's way of processing, integrating, and understanding new information. It appears that during REM sleep, the brain makes more distant neural associations that do not happen during wakefulness.[2] These nighttime changes in thinking and analyzing can easily lend themselves to altering aspects of creativity, problem solving, decision making, learning, memory consolidation, and insight. As such, sleep can provide us with a convenient second opinion about our daytime problems. Even more exciting, this nighttime mental processing can afford us the opportunity to solve problems in creative ways.

Enhanced creativity and problem solving regularly occur while we sleep.[3] It has been theorized that sleep itself can facilitate flexible reasoning and insightful behavior.[4] Throughout history, scientists, novelists, writers, artists, and inventors have solved problems while they slept. You can do the same, and we'll explain the best way for you to prime your mind so that you can make those problem-solving associative leaps.

Deirdre Barrett, a Harvard psychologist, is well known for her research into problem solving in dreams.[5] She theorizes that dreaming is essentially *active* thinking in a *different* biochemical state. While dreams may have evolved for other purposes, they can clearly also function to help us solve problems. To use a computer analogy, dreams reboot the brain, refreshing our minds for clearer thinking. Barrett believes that dreams are a rich source of practical advice from our unconscious, and they can particularly help with problems that require visual analysis and out-of-the-box thinking. She observes that since REM sleep has been around for some 220 million years,[6] the likelihood of dreams serving more than a random function is likely. It is possible that the activity of our mind during sleep may be an evolutionary-based tool. To put it another way, dreams may very well serve as a resource that we're not utilizing to their full capacity.

It's estimated that 95 percent of all dreams aren't recalled. There is some evidence that you have to actually wake up out of a dream and immediately write it down in order to recall it the next day. It also helps if you force yourself to move as little as possible upon awakening so that you don't forget your dream's content before making notes. Even a fascinating dream can disappear within seconds after you awaken unless you make a concerted effort to preserve it. Making that effort to remember is well worth the time invested, as we'll see in a moment, since recalling dreams can provide ideas that can sometimes make you rich and famous.

Capital isn't so important in business. Experience isn't so important. You can get both these things. What is important is ideas.

—HARVEY S. FIRESTONE,

founder of Firestone Tire and Rubber Co.

HOW TO SOLVE PROBLEMS WHILE SLEEPING

To fully capitalize on the benefits of sleep, some researchers even advise an earlier bedtime if a problem is looming.[7] They suggest that you mull over the problem (without getting stressed out about it) prior to sleep. Stress will keep you from sleeping, so it's advisable to purposefully relax your mind before contemplating your problem.

Unfortunately, nighttime brain chemistry isn't conducive to retaining information that pops into your mind during dreams. If ideas or solutions are in your consciousness immediately upon awakening, it's imperative that you record them right away. Experienced practitioners of so-called "dream mining" recommend writing down all dream data, including random, unrelated, and nonsensical material, since it might make sense after further analysis, in a different context, or at a later time.[8]

New memories are stored in the hippocampus, and long-term memories are stored in the neocortex. During sleep, memories move from the hippocampus to the neocortex, and as they make this transition, they are *reordered* and structurally transformed.[9] This consolidating process sometimes allows a dreamer to gain insight into difficult problems.

Although it may be unconscious, your brain is still working offline on many of the things that you experienced during the day. You can rely on the different chemical state of sleep, free from the distractions, biases, and concerns of wakefulness, to produce highly useful solutions for your career—provided that you capture them on paper as soon as you wake up in the morning or in the middle of the night. That one-dollar notebook by your bed may prove to be the source of a million-dollar idea.[10]

If you can dream it, you can do it.

—Disney employee TOM FITZGERALD (1980)

DREAM SUCCESS STORIES

In 1787 William Blake had a dream in which his brother instructed him in the engraving process. Shortly thereafter, Blake developed an improved method of engraving relief plates. His innovation employed a special coating for copper plates, which made the process easier and faster. His fame as an engraver is largely attributed to a set of twenty-one copperplate etchings illustrating the book of Job in the Old Testament. Today, he is widely considered one of the most inspired and original English painters, and some of this success can be directly attributed to insights he received in the dream state.

The inventor of the sewing machine, Elias Howe, got the idea of how to make the needle work in the apparatus from a nightmare about cannibals. In his dream the cannibals were brandishing spears that resembled the needle and needle hole he eventually designed. The dream prompted him to shift his focus away from a needle that threaded through the middle to one where the hole was at the upper end. His invention revolutionized the garment industry, and he died a multimillionaire in 1867. In 2004 he was inducted into the United States National Inventors Hall of Fame. Not bad for a man who was inspired by a dream!

> Let us learn to dream.
>
> —FRIEDRICH A. KEKULÉ, German chemist

Friedrich Kekulé, the principal founder of the theory of chemical structures, had two dreams that were destined to change his life. In the first he was amazed to see atoms dancing about, linked to one another. He woke up and immediately began to sketch what he saw. His second vision occurred when he was struggling to determine the chemical structure of benzene. During a brief nap, he saw a serpent twisted into a circle, biting its own tail (fig. 2). Upon awakening, he realized that benzene must be structured similarly, in a ring. The field of organic chemistry sprang from this insight.[11]

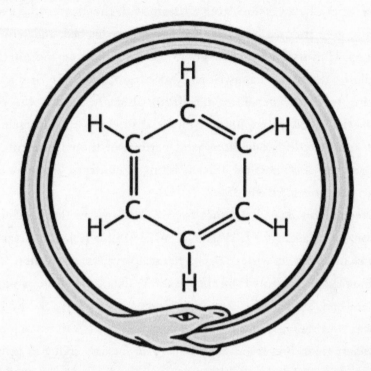

A combination of the ouroboros image and the benzene structural diagram. Kekulé claimed that the structure of benzene appeared to him in a dream that included a snake eating its tail. (Image courtesy Devlin M. Gualtieri)

We hope you're starting to see the value of keeping pen and paper by your bedside! But there's even more. Mary Shelley's *Frankenstein* was the result of a dream she had in the summer of 1816, while staying at Lord Byron's villa. At the urging of Byron, she wrote her dream down and expanded it into a novel-length manuscript. An enormous literary success, the book was published in 1818, when she was just twenty-one.

Another example of the sleeping brain helping solve a problem comes from the German pharmacologist Otto Loewi. In 1921 it wasn't known whether transmission across synapses (the space between nerve cells) was electrical or chemical. Loewi claimed that the idea for the experiment that answered this question came to him during sleep. Interestingly, he awakened from a dream with the idea for the experiment, jotted it down on a piece of paper near his bed, and returned to sleep. Unfortunately, when he awoke the following morning, his middle-of-the-night handwriting was illegible! To his dismay, he couldn't recall the details of the dream. Luckily, he had the same dream the following night, and rather than risk losing it again, he went straight to his laboratory and performed the experiment. The discovery of the chemical transmission of electrical impulses won Loewi the Nobel Prize in 1936.

Dreams also helped the first female African-American self-made millionaire, Madam C. J. Walker (1867–1919). She had a dream in which a man told her what to put on her scalp to treat an infection. Later recalling the ingredients from the dream, Walker created the salve. The Madam C. J. Walker Manufacturing Company was born, and by 1914 she was worth more than a million dollars.

Robert Louis Stevenson racked his brain for days trying to devise a new plot, at which point he fell into an exhausted sleep and dreamed the entire story for *The Strange Case of Dr. Jekyll and Mr. Hyde*. He described his dream as occurring "in that small theatre of the brain which we keep brightly lit all night long." Other famous works of art inspired by dreams include Salvador Dalí's *Persistence of Memory*, Henri Rousseau's *The Dream*, and Jasper Johns's *American Flag*.[12]

Paul McCartney admitted that "Yesterday" came to him fully formed in a dream. One night he dreamed he heard a classical string ensemble playing the melody. Fortunately for all of us, there was an upright piano next to his bed. He quickly played it, and the acclaimed song was born. He was initially worried that it was a copy of a song he had heard before but soon realized it was, indeed, an original. It has been pointed out that had the piano not been in close proximity, he might have quickly forgotten the melody. Again, this is strong evidence of how vital it is to record your dream inspirations without delay.

Other recent dreamers who achieved success as a result of their nighttime visions include Jack Nicklaus, James Cameron, and Stephenie Meyer. Nicklaus, who is considered one of the greatest golfers of all time, endured a slump in 1964, but one night, in a dream, he *saw* a new way of holding the club. The new technique worked spectacularly and propelled him back to the top of the golf world. "I feel kind of foolish admitting it," he said, "but it really happened in a dream." In 1995, James Cameron's *Avatar* sprung from an epic dream. Luckily, Cameron felt it worthwhile to take notes about this particular dream. Released in 2009, the film has grossed over $1.69 billion. Last but not least, twenty-nine-year-old stay-at-home mom Stephenie Meyer was an unpublished writer with no obvious interest in writing about vampires. One night she had a vivid dream about a vampire who was captivated by the scent of an average girl. Based on that dream, she went on to write the *Twilight* series. Her net worth is now estimated to exceed $170 million.

In a 2009 commencement address at the University of Michigan, Google cofounder Larry Page credited dreams with helping him get his start. He had a dream about cataloging the entire Web, and that eventually led to the world's most successful search engine.

Kelly Clarkson, who rose to fame after appearing on *American Idol*, confessed that she has a hard time falling asleep because new songs keep running through her head. She reportedly composes songs while drifting off to sleep but finds herself compelled to get out of bed to write down her ideas before she forgets them. She does this so often that it causes her sleep difficulties. "The moment a song comes to me, I have to get it out," she said. "That's why I have a hard time sleeping, because a lot of those times are at night."

We could add innumerable additional examples to support our point about the value of mining your dreams for success. As these anecdotes clearly demonstrate, you can sometimes solve professional and artistic problems in your sleep, and in many cases the solutions that your dream world provides are light-years ahead of what the conscious mind could discover on its own.[13]

LEARNING PHYSICAL SKILLS WHILE ASLEEP

A research study demonstrated that speed on a finger-tapping test can improve with practice, and that substantial *additional* improvement is realized following a night of sleep.[14] Admittedly, you may not be that excited about improving speed on a finger-tapping test, but these tests are routinely used to draw inferences about physical motor skills. The larger finding of this study is quite noteworthy, especially for anyone who has to perform physical tasks on the job, such as typing, focusing a camera, driving a vehicle, and so on. The conclusion that your performance of motor skill tasks can be optimized with sleep has powerful real-world implications. It may be that athletic performance, such as a golf swing or fencing thrust, depends as much on *sleeping after practice* as it does on the practice itself. The same could be said for musical skills, such as playing a violin or guitar.

A related study found that when subjects are instructed to dream about performing a motor skill that, too, can help them, especially if they succeed in dreaming about doing the task. The study involved asking participants to dream about tossing coins into a cup. Those who dreamed about the task showed significant improvement in their real-life coin tossing abilities, more so than those who did not dream about it.[15] This raises the possibility of cultivating skills during sleep.

Still another recent study tested the ability of sleep to help people solve problems. Subjects who slept were able to solve a greater number of difficult problems than those who didn't sleep, and they also found hidden rules even though they were never told that a hidden shortcut existed. However, no difference was observed in any of the groups when it came to solving easy problems. The authors concluded that sleep facilitates problem solving for more difficult problems that require a broader search for solutions.[16]

> I think sleep is involved in rehearsing, restructuring, and reclassifying
> our existing world view to allow us to function better.
>
> —DR. ROBERT STICKGOLD

It is clear that sleep is an amazing resource available to all of us. Whether we are napping, sleeping through the night, waking, or entering the groggy presleep state, sleep in its many forms can provide us with advantages in perspective, creativity, insight, learning, and problem solving. It is time that the ubiquitous myth of sleeping less to work more is dispelled. Additionally, sleeping more may end up providing the competitive advantage shared by the well rested, and tapping into this unique state of mind may serve to enhance numerous aspects of our lives. To be more effective in the boardroom, you may want to spend more time in the bedroom.

PART TWO

SLEEPING FOR PROFIT

CHAPTER SIX

STRANGE BEDFELLOWS

Cannot the laborers understand that by overworking themselves they exhaust their own strength and that of their progeny, that they are used up and long before their time come to be incapable of any work at all, that absorbed and brutalized by this single vice they are no longer men but pieces of men, that they kill within themselves all beautiful faculties, to leave nothing alive and flourishing except the furious madness for work.

—Paul Lafargue, *The Right to Be Lazy* (1907)

Almost 50 percent of American workers suffers from a sleep disorder.[1] A significant number of them are so sleep deprived that they're wandering through the day more impaired than if they were intoxicated.[2] Their sleep problems are chronic,[3] which means they may never enjoy a normal day and can't even remember what it feels like to be refreshed by a good night's sleep. But give these workers the sleep they *need* to succeed, and they will feel like new people. Their productivity will climb and they will become mentally and physically healthier.[4]

GETTING THE SLEEP YOU NEED

Although experts recommend seven to nine hours of sleep daily, American adults are clearly working more and sleeping less. Thirty percent of civilian employed adults in the United States sleep less than six hours per night.[5] It's estimated that current sleep deprivation among workers is worse today than it has ever been in the past. The average American works 1,949 hours each year.[6] In comparison, for example, a thirteenth-century peasant worked only 1,620 hours. Although today a standard workweek is forty hours, in the Unites States 85.8 percent of males and 66.5 percent of females work more than forty hours.

In all of this frenzy to work, what is happening to our sleep? Unfortunately, it's getting squeezed out of our lives. Each year we work more and sleep less.[7] This decline in sleep time is unsustainable—for individuals and organizations alike. Research has repeatedly demonstrated that employees who lack sleep perform worse than their well-rested counterparts.[8] In 2011, the Annual Sleep in America Poll conducted by the National Sleep Foundation revealed that almost two-thirds (63 percent) of Americans are not getting an adequate amount of sleep during the workweek. Most respondents felt that they required about seven and a half hours of sleep to feel their best, yet they admitted to getting only about six hours and fifty-five minutes of sleep on typical weeknights. About 15 percent of adults between ages nineteen and sixty-four and 7 percent of those between ages thirteen and eighteen said they slept less than six hours on weeknights. What is troubling is that it has been demonstrated that individuals sleeping less than seven hours a night for a couple of weeks have impairment levels similar to people who have not slept at all for one to two days.

The first step toward getting the sleep you need is recognizing that there is a deficit to begin with. Once we have recognized this need, we can take steps to rectify the problem.

Sleep Deprivation Is a
Public Health Concern

New Jersey has instituted Maggie's Law for those who have had no sleep for twenty-four hours prior to an accident. Maggie's Law states that a sleep-deprived driver qualifies as a reckless driver who can be convicted of vehicular homicide. It's named in honor of Maggie McDonnell, a twenty-year-old college student who was killed when a driver who later admitted he hadn't slept for thirty hours crossed three lanes of traffic and struck her car head-on in 1997.

A Florida man is serving a thirty-year sentence for running a truck into cars stopped at a red light. Three people were killed. He had been awake for thirty hours straight prior to the crash.

HOW TO IMPROVE YOUR CONCENTRATION

Concentration and mental focus are critical for job success. If you could improve this one factor, you would be ahead of the game.

Employees that are sleep deficient are cognitively and physically deficient, both on and off the clock. In one state where we worked, the government adopted a policy of zero tolerance for falling asleep at work for all state employees. The state Employee Assistance Program (EAP) then declared that it would be necessary to educate all state employees about sleep. They hired us to do this educating. We soon learned that employers spend more on health care costs for employees with sleep problems than for those who sleep well. Recent studies demonstrate that four to six hours of sleep nightly results in a progressive, cumulative deterioration in neurobehavioral function, including cognitive performance, rational memory, innovation, creativity, mood, short-term memory, and vigilance.[9] Work and relationship problems increase stress levels, which in turn can exacerbate sleep problems.[10]

On the other hand, there is little doubt that good sleep positively affects work performance and working relationships. With adequate sleep, employees have less difficulty concentrating, communicating, and learning. With adequate sleep, there is also an associated increase in problem-solving abilities. Getting enough sleep will help you have a better mood, causing you to be less prone to emotional outbursts and other relationship-destroying behaviors that can have disruptive effects on the entire organization you work for.

In order to improve mental concentration on the job, it is essential to first understand that sleep deprivation makes it hard to perceive how debilitated you are. There's a profound lack of insight with sleepiness; that is, a sleepy person remains largely unaware of any deficits, even significant ones. This lack of insight results in people working and driving while they're dangerously sleepy. A simple understanding of this largely universal lack of recognition on the part of the sleepy individual should prompt friends, family, and employers to raise awareness and intervene when impairment from sleepiness is suspected.

> For every hour of sleep we lose, we are also losing an IQ point—and those points can only be replenished through sleep. Theoretically, when a multitude of employees are sleep deprived, one can assume that the collective IQ of the organization is compromised.
> —STANLEY COREN, University of British Columbia (1999)

PRODUCTIVITY

At one time or another, most everyone has had a bad night of sleep and struggled through the following day. That said, a recent study suggests that people with sleep disturbances experience a significant decline in productivity. Researchers found that response times and overall productivity continued to decline the longer each participant was awake. A Canadian study estimates that employees with insomnia lost an incredible twenty-eight days of work productivity annually due to sleepiness.[11]

The good news is that you can increase productivity by fixing sleep problems. In a 2008 National Sleep Foundation survey, rested workers were more likely than sleepy workers to engage in productive interactions at work, were more patient with others, and experienced less trouble prioritizing and organizing work. In a 2010 survey of one thousand office workers by Philips Consumer Lifestyle, Americans who got adequate sleep on a consistent basis were more productive than their sleep-deprived colleagues. They enjoyed the following advantages of getting sufficient sleep.

- 85 percent of office workers surveyed felt they were more productive if they had enough sleep.
- 64 percent of office workers surveyed found that adequate sleep meant their day began on a high note.

DON'T BE A WORKAHOLIC

The term *workaholic* first appeared in the English language in 1968.[12] This fact in and of itself should tell you something about how contemporary society is moving toward madness. Overworking is a respectable *addiction* in our culture. Workaholics, type A personalities, and the overly ambitious worker or executive may desire to work longer hours, thereby requiring their brains to be active more hours of the day.[13] This practice of working longer may afford the illusion of success and peak performance, but it is not the same as working hard. Research has linked longer work hours with weaker mental skills and overall ineffectiveness, which can be attributable to a lack of sleep. A study of 2,214 middle-aged workers concluded that employees working more than fifty-five hours a week had *poorer* mental skills than their forty-hour-work week counterparts. Yet needing sleep, not workaholism, is a stigma in America. Dr. Daniel Amen, a brain imaging specialist, makes the analogy that the brain is a computer that needs to shut down on a regular basis to prevent cognitive fatigue. Overwork also takes a toll on the body. A research study that tracked seven thousand workers over more than a decade found that working eleven hours a day increased the risk of heart attack by 67 percent.[14]

> When you find depression, even when you find anxiety, when you scratch the surface, 80 to 90 percent of the time you find a sleep problem as well.
>
> —BRAD WOLGAST, University of Delaware psychologist

REDUCE STRESS

It is well known that stress interferes with good sleep. One of the greatest sources of stress, ironically, is worry about work issues and problems.[15] Stress impacting sleep is one of the most common complaints seen in a sleep clinic practice, with most stress reportedly emanating from the work environment. Studies show that stress and the social situation at work are strongly linked to disturbed sleep and impaired awakening.[16]

The relationship between sleep and stress is bidirectional. This means that sleep loss causes stress and stress causes sleep loss. While most jobs are associated with at least some stress, if the level of stress is so high that it is interfering with sleep, you may need to take action to decrease the stress or improve sleep. Many stress management programs may help you begin to better tolerate unavoidable stress at work. In addition, you should consider many of the ideas we discuss in this book to help preserve your sleep even if your stress level can't be decreased. Clearly it would be better to reduce stress at work. But if that isn't possible, improving sleep will serve to increase your tolerance of the stress.

> The fact is, when we look at well-rested people, they're operating at a different level than people trying to get by on one to two hours less nightly sleep.
>
> —DR. MERRILL MITLER, National Institutes of Health

EIGHTY PERCENT OF SUCCESS IS SHOWING UP FULLY RESTED

We're paraphrasing Woody Allen here because what he said is so true. According to Allen, who has made this point numerous times, "80 percent of success is showing up." But what does this mean for you, a person who wants more quality sleep and more success as a result of it? Well, when you get right down to it, this is probably the most important advice we can offer: if you wish to be a success, you need to show up for work refreshed from a good night's sleep. Even more important, you have to show up having had good sleep for the past week. Unless you do that, you're playing with half your brain tied behind your back.[17]

> Even moderate sleep deprivation has an effect similar to having a few too many alcoholic beverages, resulting in clumsiness, impaired judgment, and an inability to handle complex tasks.

But how do we accomplish this vital goal? It is helpful to begin by understanding that workers who do not get the appropriate amounts of sleep increase expenses for absenteeism as well as insurance costs.[18] Even if sleep-deprived employees go to work, productivity and revenue are still lost because these employees are not functioning, a condition known as "presenteeism." Research published in April 2012 by a European health consulting firm revealed the following statistics about employees:

- Almost one-half had just seven or less hours of sleep per night.
- Approximately one-quarter reported that they still felt exhausted even after sleeping.
- Approximately 5 percent slept less than five hours per night.

Compared to other employees, those with a high-risk sleeping pattern had a rate of absenteeism ten times higher than those without such a pattern, according to the survey. With myriad other problems reported, the research concluded that as much as one-third of a typical organization's workforce could be adversely affected by sleep deprivation.

Let's stop right here. Imagine you're at work. Now look to the left, and look to the right. One-third of the people you see are sleep deprived. Do you know what this means for your career? It means that a sizable percentage of your colleagues, supervisors, and managers are in a state of decreased functioning. It means that you, too, may be one of the people afflicted by this mental and physical decline. But more importantly, it means that if you figure out a way to get more sleep, you will boost yourself into the upper tier of functionality on the job. You will perform better and accomplish more. If you're self-employed, for example, you can expect to do better than your competition, develop better business plans, and win more customers.

Research has demonstrated that worksite programs can help employees get better sleep and be more productive.[19] To effectively lower presenteeism, employers can provide education, preferably as part of orientation as well as on an ongoing basis. Many employees don't know these programs exist. Even if you think you know enough about sleep, it does help to listen to other people, especially those who have been trained to help with specific issues—so take advantage of such programs your employer might offer.

REDUCE WORKPLACE ACCIDENTS

Studies show that work-related accidents don't happen randomly. They tend to occur between midnight and six in the morning and between two and four in the afternoon, when people are sleepiest. Sleep-deprived workers significantly increase the risk of accidents and injuries. Long work hours combined with poor sleep characteristics are synergistically associated with an increased risk of workplace injury, accident, and error.[20] Before the Industrial Revolution, a single individual generally controlled no more than two horsepower, usually in the form of two horses. If the driver fell asleep, the horses stayed awake and usually no harm was done. But today, the actions of a single individual can affect everyone in an office, a building, or even a city. The *Exxon Valdez* oil spill, the Space Shuttle *Challenger* explosion, and the Chernobyl and Bhopal disasters have all been attributed to sleep deprivation. While these tragedies capture international attention, the fact is that *all* businesses are affected by sleep loss, sleepiness, and fatigue that do not make headlines. Employers have sleep-deprived and fatigued employees negotiating sensitive contracts, producing products, managing money, and driving trucks. These employees are compromised, as are the businesses they operate. When adequate sleep improves clarity of thinking and response times, the result can be serious social and financial advantages for your business that could figure in the billions. Common sense dictates that greater attention be paid to managing poor sleep and reducing excessive work hours to improve safety at the workplace. Rather than pushing for longer work hours, managers should be focusing on more productive and safer work time.

Many jobs are likely to involve dangerous situations where accidents can be fatal. Driving trucks, operating heavy machinery, and working forklifts are some examples where sleepiness can have catastrophic consequences. Sleep deprivation elevates accident risk in the workplace.[21] Twenty percent of all vehicle crashes are linked to drowsy driving.[22] Hours of service rules for commercial drivers were recently updated by the Federal Motor Carrier Safety Administration to compensate for both the fatigue of long hours and the negative effects of sleeping outside our circadian phase.

In the transportation industry, the consequences are far-reaching for a wide variety of sectors, from pilots to air traffic controllers to truckers. In fact, sleepiness surpasses drugs and alcohol as the single most identifiable and preventable cause of accidents in all modes of transportation. Roadway crashes are the top cause of work-related deaths in the United States, and drowsy driving is often a factor. Sleepy drivers are a problem for all of us since we all use the roads. In the United States about three hundred thousand people fall asleep while driving every day. Their crashes result in sixty thousand injuries and eight thousand deaths per year.

Hospital interns working twenty-four hours had a 61 percent increased risk of stabbing themselves with a needle or scalpel. Their risk of a car crash increased 168 percent. Shift work is a time-honored tradition for hospital nurses. But research suggests people tend to be less alert and focused during the last four hours of a twelve-hour shift. This raises special concerns for jobs related to public health and safety. Starting in 2004, Dr. Charles Czeisler, a professor and sleep expert at Harvard Medical School, published a series of reports in medical journals based on a study of 2,700 first-year medical residents. These young men and women worked grueling shifts as long as thirty hours twice a week. Dr. Czeisler's research was groundbreaking in its revelation of the remarkable public health risk that resulted from sleep debt. Reportedly, one out of five first-year residents admitted to making fatigue-related mistakes that resulted in patient injury. One in twenty admitted to making a fatigue-related mistake that resulted in the death of a patient. One related study found that medical interns made 35.9 percent more serious medical errors during extended-duration shifts than during shifts of less than sixteen hours.

Many businesses are now working 24/7. As a result, shift work is an inevitable aspect of modern society. It has been shown that shift workers get two hours less sleep when they sleep during the day compared to when they sleep at night. Unfortunately for shift workers, humans are nocturnal sleepers. We sleep better at night. Shift workers are trying to stay awake when physiologically their bodies want to sleep. Then they try to sleep when their bodies say it is time to be awake. Often shift workers revert back to a nighttime sleep schedule on their days off. This keeps their circadian rhythms from ever adjusting to a set schedule. But that may not matter. Light is what sets the clock, and if you get off work after the sun has risen, your internal clock will be set to a daytime schedule.

International travelers are often in a time zone that's out of phase with their physiology. If they stay in the new time zone long enough, their rhythms will adapt. This is because the whole environment is working to adjust their rhythms: the sun comes up in the morning and sets at night; breakfast, lunch, and dinner are served at local times, not home time. Business travelers in new time zones should try to arrange to have meetings when they are at their circadian peak, which can give them an advantage over the people from the local time zone. For the shift worker, however, the environment in their own time zone is always working against their adjusting to these rhythms. The sun comes up at bedtime and sets when it is time to wake up. Additionally, there is no taboo about calling someone who you know is a shift worker at two in the afternoon. We would never call our friends or colleagues at two in the morning just to chat or ask a trivial favor. People come to the door, children are up playing, lawns are being mowed, and life can be noisy.

Shift work puts stress on individuals in other ways. There is often a disconnect between spouses and other family members. The night worker often misses family activities and accomplishments such as recitals or graduations. Work environments may be designed for comfort rather than productivity. We once visited a 911 operator's office. It had very comfortable chairs, the lighting was recessed and dim, and the room was cold and quiet. This was a great environment for sleeping, not dealing with life-threatening emergencies.

MANAGING SLEEP AT WORK

Corporate America has smoking policies, lunch breaks, coffee breaks, maternity and sick leave policies—but virtually no acknowledgment of the biological need for sleep. Which raises the question: Are employers understanding and using sleep to their advantage? It is apparent that sleep problems are pervasive, but their effect on the workplace and our personal performance in the workplace is enormous and underestimated. Most employers can't monitor an employee's bedtime or ensure sleep quality, but some are taking the research seriously by managing sleep through educational and support activities, as well as by fostering a corporate culture that doesn't promote sleepless machismo. Because poor sleep quality can reduce an individual's productivity and increase the prevalence of illness, awareness and targeted interventions are becoming increasingly important for businesses. Data supports the value of worksite interventions and education, and studies have demonstrated that group education on sleep hygiene, along with individual behavioral training, can significantly improve the quality of sleep for workers.

Cost-conscious corporations provide sleep awareness programs and seminars for their employees, even incorporating them into employee orientation programs. The seminars range from hour-long lectures to multiweek courses that educate, raise awareness, and provide solutions to sleep problems. With corporate sponsorship, successful implementation of such a proactive approach will increase the bottom line through reduced absenteeism, increased retention, superior job satisfaction, higher productivity, and more efficient performance. Forward-thinking corporations are successfully utilizing education on sleep hygiene, insomnia reduction techniques, and sleep apnea management.

ADJUSTING EMPLOYEE SCHEDULES

Beyond helping individual sleep-deprived employees, employers and managers should ensure that corporate scheduling is not contributing to sleep deprivation. Scheduling should aim to limit the number of hours worked, maximize sleep opportunity, and minimize the risk of employee fatigue during work. There are several approaches to optimizing work schedules. One proven strategy is to start work later in the day. Each extra hour before the start of work results in employees obtaining twenty minutes of extra sleep time.[23] Not only will employees be more productive, they'll also be grateful for the extra sleep.

Dr. Charles Czeisler, the Harvard Medical School sleep expert, recommends that employees working the night shift not work more than four or five days in a row. Some research also supports that night shifts that begin after midnight allow workers to get more sleep and experience less fatigue than shifts that start between 8:00 p.m. and midnight. Companies can address the problem by offering orientation programs, giving employees flexibility in making their schedules, reducing shift rotations, and providing on-site child care.

Special attention needs to be paid to long-term shift workers. These employees may easily adapt to a night shift when they're in their twenties, but for some people, shift work becomes physically and emotionally more difficult with age. About 25 percent of nineteen- to thirty-five-year-olds can't sleep well during the day, and more than 40 percent of fifty-five- to sixty-four-year-olds have the same problem. A new area of research is showing that some individuals may be genetically unable to work the night shift. A particular form of the circadian gene, PER3, makes it very difficult for some people to sleep during the day.

Workloads should be also prioritized so that work requiring the highest concentration is conducted at the beginning of the shift to ensure safety and accuracy. In shift work, a worker is usually performing lowest during the last three hours of the shift.

CORPORATE CULTURE

The culture of the American corporation must acknowledge sleep health and adapt to reflect the recent scientific research in the field of sleep medicine. Corporate America can no longer condone a culture where excessive overwork and overtime are encouraged and sleep is discouraged. Fatigue is neither a weakness nor a vice—it is a physiological vulnerability.

The employee who's the first to arrive every morning and the last to leave every night is no longer the corporate role model on the trajectory to success. The formula for success is not a matter of working more hours and sleeping less. Sufficient sleep permits higher functioning on all levels: personal, social, and vocational. Rather, the clear-thinking, ethical, and creative employee is the new corporate role model destined for success. This employee has a realistic understanding of time management and will reap the cognitive, emotional, and physical benefits of sufficient sleep. Therefore the successful individual prioritizes and manages sleep, as does the successful organization.

SLEEPING YOUR WAY TO THE TOP

As sleep research continues, cultural changes will follow. Hours of service have already changed for truck drivers to accommodate their need for sleep. In December 2011 the Federal Aviation Administration modified flight schedules to ensure adequate time for pilots to sleep. These examples reflect a new and enlightened attitude more consistent with what sleep science is discovering about the need for sleep to prevent accidents.

Sleeping your way to the top is no longer a misnomer or reference to a roundabout way of succeeding, and you know what we mean. Instead, it is a modern motivational maxim steeped in science that can bring success to those who utilize it. Yes, the message is loud and clear: *sleep to be successful.*

Add an hour or two of sleep if you're accumulating sleep debt. Experience the changes for yourself. Because the inverse—sacrificing sleep in order to work—is inefficient: it is the equivalent of being penny wise and pound foolish. Sacrificing sleep in order to work is a discredited, false formula for success. If you want to be more productive and work more efficiently, don't cut back on sleep. Instead, eliminate time wasters: stop watching TV programs that do nothing to add to the quality of your life, learn to say no to people and causes that encroach upon your valuable time, and delegate and outsource certain activities.

Think of all the things you can cut back on—with the exception of sleep—if you find yourself without enough hours during the day. After all, the *quality* of hours is more important than their *quantity*. A well-rested person can accomplish much more in fewer hours than a sleep-deprived person can.

Historically, sleep and work have been unlikely bed partners. However, raised awareness and the education of individual employees and corporate America can put work and sleep in bed together.

The Talmud states: "An unexamined dream is like an unopened letter."

The prevailing attitude in our society is that you can't be successful, climb to the top, stay ahead of the competition, and lead the pack without sacrificing sleep. There is an entrenched belief that sleepiness is somehow associated with laziness, lack of motivation, and the absence of work ethic. But compelling scientific evidence strongly disproves this attitude. We now have proof that sufficient sleep leads to high levels of functioning, success, and good health, both for the individual and the organization.

Quite literally, sleep improves every element of workplace success and personal success. An estimated 36 million Americans believe that sleeplessness harms their job performance in such areas as handling stress, making decisions, and solving problems. This sleeplessness is a physical and psychological stumbling block. The gain in efficiency, creativity, innovation, clarity of thought, memory, and overall performance that sleep brings far outweighs any benefit of mindlessly adding hours to your day by subtracting sleep hours. The equation is new; the math is simple: adding sleep adds quality. By sleeping soundly and sufficiently, a person is more likely to do everything better and feel better while doing it.

CHAPTER SEVEN

STAYING POWER

I can know all the plays like the back of my hand. I can lift all the
weights in the world. But if I get five, six hours of sleep, I'm going
to have that doubt in my head and that sluggish nature, and you
can't have that when you're trying to block these elite guys.
I'd absolutely say sleep is a weapon.

—Kyle Long, *Chicago Tribune* (2015)

Babe Ruth may have a reputation for being the bad boy of baseball, but
the truth about him is much more interesting. His second wife, Claire
Hodgson, badgered him to sleep more.[1] Apparently Hodgson knew the
value of sleep even if Ruth didn't. Her advice, which the legendary baseball player followed to the letter, enabled the slugger to accomplish more
in the latter part of his career than most players achieve in their lives.[2]
For example, in one of his last games, on May 30, 1935, he hit three
home runs.

Nowhere else is the need for peak performance more obvious than in
sports. Athletes must demonstrate, very publicly, their best efforts over
and over again. It is increasingly more apparent that adequate sleep is as
important as practice in achieving that performance.

On the night before the seventh game of the 2011 Stanley Cup,
Dr. Charles Czeisler received an emergency phone call from the Boston

Bruins team doctor. The Bruins hadn't won this prize for thirty-nine years. The doctor wanted to know if there was anything that could help equalize the home court advantage held by the Canucks. He knew that Dr. Czeisler had worked with other sports teams and even musicians such as Mick Jagger. The game was to start at 5:00 p.m. Vancouver time. The Bruins had a practice scheduled at 10:30 a.m. Dr. Czeisler suggested they skip practice and take a nap instead. *Skip practice?* The team doctor couldn't believe his ears. But Dr. Czeisler pointed out that when it was 10:30 a.m. in Vancouver, it was 1:30 p.m. in Boston, a good time for an East Coast team to be napping. The Bruins followed his advice, canceled practice, and took to their beds for the prescribed nap. Later that evening, they defeated the Canucks and won the Stanley Cup.[3]

This story illustrates how finding a competitive edge can require an athlete to look in unusual places. As you can imagine, maintaining a career as a professional athlete is physically and psychologically demanding. Many successful athletes now understand the performance-enhancing benefits of sufficient sleep and the competitive edge that it provides.[4] Apolo Anton Ohno averages eight to eight and a half hours of sleep each night. Tom Brady reportedly hits the hay between 8:30 p.m. and 9:00 p.m., citing plenty of sleep as a strategy he utilizes to play the game he loves for as long as possible.[5] Do these power players know something we don't?

As we've already seen, insufficient sleep does a number on our cognitive and physical functioning. Reaction time is slowed; thinking is more emotional and less rational. An athlete needs to make decisions instantly. A pause of even microseconds may make the difference between a gold medal and no medal.

> Asking athletes to play on minimal sleep is the same as asking them
> to play with one hand tied behind their back.
>
> —DR. CHARLES CZEISLER

When we're sleep deprived, the brain handles information differently, in part because the amygdala, which is responsible for emotion, is 60 percent more active. Rather than process data primarily with the logical cortex, the brain tends to shunt information through this older, less rational part.[6]

Insufficient sleep also decreases testosterone levels. A recent study showed that even moderate sleep restriction reduces daytime testosterone 10 to 15 percent.[7] Levels were lowest from early afternoon to early evening, times important for many athletes. Testosterone is critical for male sexual behavior and reproduction, and also has important beneficial effects on muscle mass and strength, adiposity, bone density, cognition, and well-being.[8]

In addition to testosterone, there are other negative endocrine changes associated with sleep deprivation: after only one week of sleep restriction, young healthy males experienced glucose levels that were no longer normal, indicating a rapid deterioration of the body's ability to handle metabolic tasks.[9] This reduced ability to deal with glucose is similar to that found in the elderly.

SLEEP EXTENSION

An effective tool for improving performance is sleep extension. Put simply, this entails *sleeping more than your customary amount of sleep time*. Sleep extension improves athletic recovery. That is, it helps athletes regain muscle strength after a game or a workout in the gym.[10]

How much is enough? It varies among individual athletes. Steve Nash of the Lakers shoots for ten hours per night and naps every game day. Basketball star Derrick Rose takes a three-hour nap before night games. Golf pro Michelle Wie sleeps twelve hours when possible and admits to not feeling good with less than ten hours. Some sleep studies have experimented with a ten-hour sleep extension. Fifteen healthy college students were tested to see if such a sleep extension had value. Now, mind you, these weren't students with sleep problems: they were already sleeping well *before* the study. The intervention consisted of asking them to sleep *as much as possible during the test.* The results? *Extended sleep led to substantial improvements in reaction time, as well as improvements in other markers of health, such as alertness and mood.*[11]

In another sleep extension study, eleven healthy men from the Stanford University men's varsity basketball team were instructed to get as much sleep as possible, with the requirement being that they sleep a minimum of ten hours per night. The results were impressive: when they got more sleep, they had faster sprint times and improved shooting accuracy, with free-throw percentage increasing by 9 percent. Their three-point field goal percentage went up by a significant 9.2 percent. And their reaction time decreased (a good thing). In short, they had quicker reflexes after getting the extra sleep. Such demonstrations of improvements following sleep extension suggest that *peak performance can occur only when an athlete optimizes sleep time.*

What does this say for the rest of us? We believe the message is clear: *even if you think you're getting sufficient sleep, you're probably not.* If you allow yourself to sleep more, your ability to perform well in sports—and do other physical tasks—is likely to increase markedly.

> Fatigue makes cowards of us all.
>
> —VINCE LOMBARDI, football coach

SLEEPING AFTER THE FACT

Memory continues to be solidified in the brain after we learn new tasks. Sleeping improves this unconscious skill acquisition process. That's one of the reasons why it's important to get a good night's sleep after learning something new. Sleep boosts memory for *facts* and also for *physical actions*. If you've been practicing your golf swing, for example, your brain will continue to work on the swing while you sleep. And when you wake up, you'll find that your game has improved.

Direct evidence for this beneficial effect of sleep was demonstrated by researchers at MIT. They recorded neuronal activity in the hippocampus of rats learning to find food in a maze. They got to the point that the researcher could tell where in the maze a rat was based on the pattern of neurons firing. When the rats were asleep, the researchers saw that they produced the same pattern of neuronal firing that had occurred during wakefulness. In effect, the rats continued to practice the task even during sleep. Sleep researcher Matthew Walker tested motor control speed by having people tap numbers in a specific sequence as quickly as possible. After twelve hours, subjects were retested. Some subjects slept during that time; others didn't. Subjects who slept showed a rather spectacular 20 percent increase in speed with 35 percent greater accuracy.[12] This increase in motor speed doesn't occur if you stay awake. In other words, in order to get this benefit—increased motor skill performance—you need to sleep.[13] It appears that the enhancement to learning occurs within twenty-four hours after learning. If you wait longer, you won't experience the enhancement that sleep offers.

Lesson from the laboratory: after learning a new skill, sleep on it. This sleep will consolidate your memory of the new skill. It will also rev up your ability to process nutrients such as glucose. Like the bionic man, you can look forward to being *better, stronger, faster*.

BANKING SLEEP

Olympic athletes nap, on average, half an hour per day.[14] Some, like Bernie Williams, love to nap just before playing a game. Boxers can often be seen napping before a bout. These precompetition naps strengthen an athlete's ability. They are "advantageous to performance," as one study put it.[15] J. J. Watt bought a bed and put it in the Houston Texans training room for napping.

In addition to taking a nap on the day of the game, banking sleep on the nights *leading up to a game* is also a good idea. Let's look at why this might be so. To examine this question, researchers decided to study one of the most grueling races, the Ultra-Trail du Mont-Blanc. In this race, runners travel from France to Italy to Switzerland and cover 103 miles. The best way to prepare? The study found that the single best tactic consisted of increasing sleep time for some nights *prior* to the race. In short, putting sleep in the bank was the winning strategy. This race was so long that some contestants stopped to take a nap *during* the contest! But that wasn't the best strategy: contestants who stopped to nap during the race lost time and energy. The winning approach was to bank sleep *before the race*.[16]

Can you use the same technique? Certainly, and it's easy to do. For instance, any businessperson can use this same strategy before an important conference by getting extra sleep on the nights leading up to the meeting. When you have an event of any type coming up, discipline yourself so that you manage to increase sleep on a few nights prior to the event. By putting sleep in the bank, you'll be giving yourself a competitive edge.[17]

> Basketball players who practice sleep extension—sleeping as much as they want—run faster, enjoy quicker reflexes, shoot more accurately, achieve a better free throw percentage, and attain an increased three-point field goal percentage.

BENEFITS OF SLEEP FOR ATHLETES

Did Babe Ruth hit more home runs because his second wife urged him to sleep more? While that might be hard to prove with any degree of confidence, we certainly can quantify specific benefits that athletes derive from improved sleep, corrected sleep problems, and extended sleep.

When they're allowed to sleep as much as they wish, athletes experience substantial improvements in reaction time.[18] The same result is likely to occur with a truck driver, an airline pilot, or a mom driving a minivan, for whom reaction time is a critical driving skill. Additional advantages of sleep extension should be plain to see.

> Sleep is extremely important to me. I need to rest and recover in order for the training I do to be absorbed by my body.
>
> —USAIN BOLT, Jamaican sprinter

TREATING SLEEP PROBLEMS

You'll do much better in any competition if you take care of sleep problems. This includes insomnia, apnea, sleepwalking, and a host of other sleep abnormalities. By getting treatment, you can fully realize the benefits of quality, sufficient sleep.

By some estimates, as many as one in three NFL players suffers from obstructive sleep apnea. In fact, the late great Reggie White died in his sleep at the age of forty-three due to conditions related to sleep apnea. Shaquille O'Neal was diagnosed with moderate obstructive sleep apnea in 2011 and has reported that treatment has left him with more energy and a greater ability to manage his weight.

To study the effect of treating obstructive sleep apnea in athletes, scientists evaluated the use of nasal positive airway pressure (PAP) therapy in skilled golfers. In addition to physical ability, golf is a game requiring a significant amount of mental skill. Golfers with apnea had a worse handicap index (a measure of golf ability) and reported being sleepier on the green. Clearly lack of sleep was impairing their mental functioning. When PAP machines corrected the apnea of these skilled golfers, they improved their handicap index by a whopping 31.5 percent! Look no further for evidence that correcting sleep problems can pay off for an athlete.

Athletes often lose sleep prior to a competition. They're only human, after all. A majority (82.1 percent) admit to staying up worrying about the game. They also have trouble falling asleep because they're going over the contest in their minds (83.5 percent) and they feel nervous (43.8 percent).[19] Again, all too human reactions. This is called a "situational," rather than a "global," problem. That is, it occurs only in a specific situation: prior to a competition. Researchers recommend that coaches help athletes learn effective ways to reduce worry and increase quality sleep prior to competition.

Mark Rosekind, a former NASA scientist now on the National Transportation Safety Board, was asked to improve the sleep of athletes at the Olympic training facility in Colorado Springs. The first thing he did was change beds, lighting, and temperature. He also reduced noise. Then he invited speed skater Apolo Ohno to try the new sleep setup. It improved Ohno's performance almost immediately. When other athletes saw his room, they became envious and wanted to know when theirs would be available.[20]

Nerves aren't the only factor causing sleep loss before competitions. Travel is also implicated. Red-eye flights and morning practices interfere with sleep. But a more subtle factor is at work here: travel through different time zones influences how an athlete performs when away from home. In 2013 researchers studied the past forty years of professional football games, comparing East Coast to West Coast teams. They employed the point spread used for betting purposes, since it takes into account all known factors that could influence the outcome of a game. Teams playing at their peak circadian times had the advantage, especially in evening games, where results were strongly in favor of West Coast teams.

Circadian rhythms strongly influence athletic performance. We perform significantly better at certain circadian times. As a quick review: body temperature starts to rise before we wake, reaches a peak in early evening, then falls during sleep, with the low temperature occurring at around four in the morning.[21] In 1983, English researchers demonstrated that circadian rhythms affect performance in trained swimmers. Subjects swam one hundred meters 2.7 seconds faster in the evening as opposed to the morning. Speed increased as body temperature increased. If you think this is a trivial result, remember that the difference between Olympic gold and silver is usually less than a second. The lesson is clear: the time *when* we do things affects *how* we do things. If two people in different circadian times are interacting, one will have an important advantage over the other.

Athletes must tap into the mind and body to an extreme degree in order to win. Successful athletes make sleep their ultimate weapon in the perpetual quest to be the best. The most important implication for you is that quality sleep can be instrumental in staying on top of your game, regardless of which game you're playing.

CHAPTER EIGHT

IF YOU'VE GOT IT, FLAUNT IT

Get at least eight hours of beauty sleep. Nine if you're ugly.

—Betty White

In Sweden a group of scientists led by Dr. John Axelsson recently investigated an intriguing question. They hoped to find out whether there was anything to the notion of beauty sleep.

They began with two known facts. First, sleep deprivation is a common condition among patients seeking medical help. Second, the human face is the main source of information for social signaling.[1] Put more simply, this means that when you get together with someone, your face is the center of their attention when they interact with you. Dr. Axelsson and his group surmised that sleep might affect facial attractiveness and, if so, it follows logically that physicians should be able to determine whether patients are sleep deprived simply by looking at them during routine office visits. Doctors who notice visible signs of sleep loss can make recommendations to improve the general health of those patients.

But Dr. Axelsson's study has even bigger implications for us. We want to know how sleep can propel us higher in our careers. More specifically, we want to know whether being more attractive has any value in the business and professional world, and, if so, if sleep can boost our attractiveness.

> Your sleep, and how you sleep, affects how other people perceive you, and probably how they treat you.
>
> —JOHN AXELSSON, sleep researcher

The short answer to the first part of the question is yes, attractiveness *does* have value in the business world. John T. Molloy, the father of image consulting, has probably done more work on this question than anyone. After conducting three decades of investigation into the issue, he concluded that things will be significantly easier for you at work if you're attractive.[2] A recent meta-analysis found that attractiveness is a signal of health, as well as an artifact of the way our brains process information.[3] The general consensus seems to be that although attractiveness may not be a *necessary* condition for success, it's certainly a factor that can help you.[4]

Axelsson began by recruiting twenty-three young adults and taking photographs of their faces when they were fully rested, with at least eight hours of sleep, and when they were sleep deprived, with only five hours sleep. He showed these pairs of portraits to sixty-five observers, asking them to rate the photos on the basis of attractiveness and health. The results confirmed the age-old notion of the value of beauty sleep: people who had sufficient sleep were consistently rated as being more attractive and healthier than their sleep-deprived selves.

BEAUTY SLEEP REALLY CAN CONTRIBUTE TO YOUR SUCCESS.

"Sleep-deprived people are perceived as less attractive, less healthy, and more tired compared with when they are well rested," Axelsson concluded.[5]

Politically correct or not, attractive people enjoy favorable treatment in many situations, both in and out of the workplace. A recent study found that advertising agencies with good-looking executives had higher revenues and faster growth than their competitors.[6] Another study from Rice University and the University of Houston concluded that managers interviewing a deformed applicant rated the applicant lower while recalling less information from the interview.[7]

The value of these studies is clear: they confirm the idea that beauty sleep really *can* contribute to your success. On an even more fundamental level, they indicate that fixing sleep problems can also make you more attractive, a conclusion confirmed by other research demonstrating that correcting sleep apnea results in people being perceived as more attractive.[8] The bottom line is that getting enough sleep will make you more attractive, and as a result you're likely to have more success in interactions with other people.

> Patients with obstructive sleep apnea are perceived to appear more alert, more youthful, and more attractive after adherent use of positive airway pressure.
>
> —DR. RONALD DAVID CHERVIN, professor of neurology

While a lack of sleep has been linked to problems such as cognitive impairment, obesity, diabetes, cancer, and immune deficiency, sleep's demonstrated effects on skin could be considered only an old wives' tale until recently. In 2013 a study of sixty women found that sleep improves skin function and reduces the ravages of aging. Commissioned by Estée Lauder, the study demonstrated that poor sleepers suffered accelerated signs of skin aging and slower recovery from environmental stressors such as ultraviolet radiation. Also noted was that good sleepers reported a significantly better self-perception of their appearance and physical attractiveness compared with poor sleepers.[9]

For me, sleep is a major thing. I don't always get it, and when I don't,
I look like I've been hit by a truck.

—GWYNETH PALTROW, actress

HOW SLEEP BEAUTIFIES SKIN

Sleep serves to maintain levels of new cell production, human growth
hormone (HGH), and testosterone. "There's something about HGH
that helps the body repair itself," Dr. Donald Greenblatt says. Director of the Strong Sleep Disorders Clinic at the University of Rochester
Medical Center, he points out that during sleep our perspiration naturally moisturizes the skin. In addition, blood flow increases to the face,
partially eradicating wrinkles.

Dr. Donna Arand, clinical director of the Kettering Sleep Disorders
Center in Dayton, Ohio, agrees that sleep deprivation can have a negative impact on a person's features. "People's eyes don't seem to be open
quite as wide," she says. "The muscles in their face are more drawn or
relaxed." She also points out that adequate sleep helps restore muscle
tone and repair the physiological degradation that occurs during the
normal workday.

The skin is particularly susceptible to the negative consequences of
sleep deprivation, such as premature aging, dermatitis, eczema, and psoriasis. Dr. Jerome Litt, an Ohio dermatologist, notes that a lack of sleep
affects the skin in a very perceptible way. The good news is that getting
sufficient sleep can have numerous positive effects on your skin.

- Sleep makes the eyes look less puffy.
- Sleep decreases cortisol, resulting in better-looking skin.
- Sleep increases human growth hormone, building and
  repairing new skin cells.

- Sleep increases collagen production, making skin look firm and young.
- Sleep increases skin hydration, making skin softer.
- Sleep boosts the immune system, preventing rashes.

> No wonder Sleeping Beauty looked so good . . . she took long naps, never got old, and didn't have to do anything but snore to get her Prince Charming.
>
> —OLIVE GREEN, author

HOW TO SLEEP FOR BEAUTY

The key point to understand when planning to sleep for beauty is that cell-tissue repair occurs primarily in stage 3 sleep. This is deep sleep, also known as slow wave sleep (SWS), which typically occurs in the first half of the night. During SWS, human growth hormone is released, so if you don't get stage 3 sleep, you won't benefit from the secretion of this skin-friendly hormone. If you look at topical antiaging formulas, they often contain growth hormone; however, topical application is ineffective.[10] If you can maintain your natural growth hormone, it will have a real effect.

True enough, you can use a moisturizer before bed, or a humidifier in your bedroom, but neither is going to be as effective as getting sufficient stage 3 sleep. Creams and makeup aren't nearly as effective as Mother Nature at making your skin look good.

> After all, beauty is a by-product of wellness.
>
> —ELLE MACPHERSON, model

CHAPTER NINE

SLEEPING WITH THE STARS

Sleep is my weapon.

—Jennifer Lopez

It's frustrating for us as sleep clinicians to hear celebrities claim that they don't need more than a few hours of sleep each night, because we know that they're wrong. The same with the life hackers who say that you can train yourself to sleep only a few hours a night. They're all doing you a disservice. In fact, anyone who tells you that you can cut back on sleep time and still be effective is feeding you nonsense.

Acclaimed sleep researcher David F. Dinges and associates performed a test in which subjects were allowed to sleep four, six, or eight hours. During the two-week study, the subjects were challenged with the psychomotor vigilance task (PVT), the same machine used to test astronauts to make sure they can do critical space jobs without loss of mental or motor accuracy.

The results were so impressive that they were published in scientific journals as well as in the *New York Times*.[1] People who got eight hours of sleep did just fine on the test, with almost no decrement in skill. But people in the four- and six-hour sleep deprivation groups suffered profound deficits in skill level, which got worse with each day. Those in the four-hour group did worse than those in the six-hour group, but both sleep-deprived groups experienced poor results.

Conclusion: six hours isn't enough sleep.

"But what about seven hours?" you ask. "I get seven hours and I'm just fine, right?"

No, even that may not be enough. Along comes another study, this one conducted by Dr. Gregory Belenky, longtime sleep researcher, and his associates at the Walter Reed Army Institute of Research. He limited subjects to seven hours of sleep, which most people think is sufficient, and he also tested them with the PVT. These subjects experienced reduced performance, too. They performed below the level of people who had sufficient sleep (eight to nine hours). Belenky concluded that their "brain operational capacity" was restricted, and that this decrease in brain function persisted "for several days after normal sleep duration" was restored.[2]

So, now you be the judge.

For our money, the sleep researchers discussed above are much more credible than high-profile people like Donald Trump claiming to need only a few hours. You might want to think twice when you hear celebrities trying to sell you on a regimen of restricted sleep. What they're really offering you is nothing more than reduced ability to solve problems, slower reaction times, decreased performance, and suboptimal functioning. That's not the way to achieve success.

We're pleased to report, however, that there are many high-profile people who get the message. They understand the value of sleep. And they use sleep to propel their careers forward. Let us tell you about a few of them.

JENNIFER LOPEZ

This singer and consummate entertainer has learned the lesson well. We're talking about the lesson that sleep experts have been teaching for years now. She treats sleep like a priority, and her results, in terms of career success, are impressive.

"I try to get eight hours a night," she says. She also confesses that she uses sleep for antiaging, considering it essential. "Sleep is my weapon," she says. "I think sometimes we get caught up in what we need to do next and forget about what are the very essential and important things in life. I treasure my time to sleep. It's just as important as eating or exercising."[3] With numerous successful songs and films to her credit, Jennifer Lopez's advice is exactly what we'd recommend.

MARC ANDREESSEN

Cofounder of Netscape, Marc Andreesen admits that he used to work into the wee hours of the morning: "I would spend the whole day wishing I could go home and go back to bed." But this super successful software engineer has changed his ways. He now aims to get at least seven and a half hours of quality sleep nightly. If he goes below six or seven hours, he feels sleepy and doesn't work at his peak level. With only four hours he feels like a zombie, as do most people. On weekends he catches up, getting twelve hours or more each night. He says this makes a big difference in clearing his mind and allowing him to get back to normalcy.

THE DALAI LAMA

Just as the pope leads Catholics, the Dalai Lama leads Tibetan Buddhists. The current Dalai Lama is Tenzin Gyatso. He and his associates lead a life of meditation, contemplation, and public service. And no one is more intent on his meditation and public service than this spiritual leader. It should come as no surprise, then, that he treats physical requirements, such as sleeping, with great respect, bordering on veneration.

"Sleep is the best meditation," the Dalai Lama says. He also sleeps about eight hours each night, sometimes as many as nine. This practice allows him to wake up completely rested and with the sharp mental clarity needed for a leader of a major religion.

> I have no trouble sleeping.
>
> —DALAI LAMA

ARIANNA HUFFINGTON

A leading journalist and cofounder of the Huffington Post, Arianna Huffington used to sleep like many a harried entrepreneur. Getting only a few hours of rest a night, she pushed herself to the limits of human endurance and found that it was a losing battle. She became so disoriented that she fell in 2007, broke her cheekbone, and needed five stitches in her right eye.

Now, at age sixty-five, she has become one of the greatest advocates of sleep science, and she used her very successful platform, the Huffington Post, to publish a continuing stream of reports from sleep experts and researchers, all written in the reader-friendly style for which her website is famous. She calls being sleep deprived "an emblem of stupidity." She views sleepless people as misguided drunks. She even does something that we, as sleep clinicians, applaud: she provides nap rooms for her employees. Now that's a place *we'd* like to work, too.

> Arianna Huffington's secret to success?
>
> "Sleep ranks number one."

JEFF BEZOS

The founder of Amazon, Jeff Bezos, is one of the most successful entrepreneurs of all time. You might think, given all the nonsense bandied about by celebrities and billionaires who would have you believe they're invincible, that to achieve his success he would have to stay up working into the wee hours.

But no! The man who single-handedly created the largest online bookstore and then parlayed Amazon into an online seller of almost everything under the sun, a constantly innovating mastermind, treats sleep with the same kid-gloves reverence that we saw the Dalai Lama gives his slumber. In fact, Bezos has been getting eight hours a night for decades. He didn't make his mark as a sleepless, harried, pressurized type-A personality and then slow down in his later years. On the contrary, he disciplined himself like a cadet in the Marines, observing a lights-out policy that allowed him to get eight hours a night of restful slumber from the very start of his career.[4] Jeff Bezos gives the lie to the celebrities and wealthy people who claim to be sleeping only a few hours a night with no mental impairment.[5]

How to Wind Down

Reading before bed (the old-fashioned way, with print) can be a relaxing yet productive way to spend time prior to sleep. It's reported that Bill Gates is a voracious reader, spending an hour each night before bedtime reading a book. Arianna Huffington doesn't like e-books in the bedroom and reads print books to relax before sleep. We recommend nonengaging nonfiction to avoid losing precious sleep time by getting caught up in a page-turning thriller. Alternately, coloring books for adults have become another pleasurable and calming bedtime option.

For bedtime reading, avoid backlit devices. The use of portable light-emitting devices at bedtime has been shown to have negative biological effects that contribute to sleep deficiency and disrupt circadian rhythms. To reduce light exposure and to limit light range, use a reading lamp with a telescoping neck and a low-watt bulb.

One 2014 study tested the effects of blue light on sleep by asking people to read either an e-book or a print book for four hours before bed. The twelve participants who read an e-book experienced later releases in melatonin (a bad result), compared with those who had read a print book. Later release of melatonin prolongs the time it takes to fall asleep, reduces the total amount of sleep, delays the timing of REM sleep, and decreases alertness the following morning. Use of light-emitting devices immediately before bedtime also increase alertness at that time, which may lead users to delay bedtime even further.[6]

GEORGE H. W. BUSH

George H. W. Bush tried his best to sleep enough to keep his mind fresh while he was in office as the president of the United States. That wasn't always easy. If you think you have troubles, take a look at his schedule during the time the United States was at war, and you'll understand why his sleep schedule was thrown off once in a while. "I have never felt a day like this in my life," he wrote in a letter the night before he ordered the bombing of Baghdad. "I am very tired. I didn't sleep well and this troubles me because I must go to the nation at nine o'clock. My lower gut hurts . . ."[7]

But after he addressed the nation, he felt much better. In fact, he was able to sleep immediately afterward. "Well, it is now 10:45 at night," he wrote. "I am about to go to bed. I did my speech to the nation at 9:00 o'clock. I didn't feel nervous about it at all. I wrote it myself. I knew what I wanted to say, and I said it . . . Just before going to bed, Cheney calls. 56 Navy planes went out. 56 came back."[8] Secretary of Defense Dick Cheney's good news heartened the president, and despite the initiation of hostilities, he was able to retire for the night at a reasonable time.

Talk about sleeping under fire! President Bush's ability to get the sleep he needed, even during war, should inspire us all. His approach is a vital lesson on how to put the day's worries aside when it's time for bed.

TOM BRADY

Most athletes have a deep appreciation for the things they have to do in order to keep fit, including watching their diet, exercising, and getting sufficient sleep. But probably no one exemplifies this dedication to living clean more than Tom Brady, one of the most successful quarterbacks in the NFL. Among his many accomplishments, he's the only quarterback to lead his team to six Super Bowls.

You might consider this another accomplishment: Brady goes to sleep between 8:30 and 9:00 every night. He says he goes to bed so early because football is his passion, and he plans his life to enable himself to keep playing the game as long as possible. "Strength training and conditioning and how I really treat my body is important to me, because there's really nothing else that I enjoy like playing football," he says. "I want to do it as long as I can."[9]

His philosophy of life—just as we have seen with the Dalai Lama—encompasses a dedication to protecting his sleep. In fact, this man, who has devoted his life to achievement on the football field, has a lot to teach us about how we, too, can choose to value sleep.

I do go to bed very early because I'm up very early. I think that the decisions that I make always center around performance enhancement, if that makes sense. So whether that's what I eat or what decisions I make or whether I drink or don't drink, it's always football centric. I want to be the best I can be every day. I want to be the best I can be every week. I want to be the best I can be for my teammates.

I love the game and I want to do it for a long time. But I also know that if I want to do it for a long time, I have to do things differently than the way guys have always done it.[10]

Joe DiMaggio was poetry in motion, and for these remarks Brady can claim the moniker "poetry in speech." Yes, it's like reading Jack Kerouac or, dare we say it, the Psalms ... *Tom Brady, you got it right.*

HOW TO SLEEP LIKE A SUCCESS

Unless they possess a rare genetic variant allowing them to get by on less than eight or nine hours, all successful people—including celebrities, businesspeople, artists, educators, politicians, homemakers, students, and retirees—need to ensure that they obtain the requisite normal amount of sleep ... and so do you.

It's all well and good to regale you with stories about high-profile people who value their sleep and who could serve as an inspiration. But without the commitment to make a change, nothing can happen. From our clinical experience, making even incremental changes is a good way to start. Put into place a few of the sleep hygiene tips from Chapter 18, or try some of the sleep suggestions you find doable. By doing so, you'll pave the way for additional progress, which will have a cumulative positive effect and move you in the right direction.

Don't expect perfection overnight. Even sleep paragons occasionally slip and make mistakes. What is required is a steady desire to move toward better sleep, and with that attitude you will make progress.

While you can do things that will certainly help with sleep, there are really no shortcuts, gimmicks, or easy solutions that guarantee sleep other than prioritizing it and committing to a healthy sleep lifestyle.

One of the most important things you can do is to take stock of your current situation: Are you a normal sleeper but not meeting your sleep needs due to habits of behavior or environment? What factors in your bedroom, in your schedule, or in your school or workplace might be disrupting your nighttime repose, and what changes can you make to optimize your sleep? Do you have insomnia? Obviously, sleep problems, signs or symptoms of a sleep disorder, or persistent sleepiness in the face of good sleep habits and sufficient sleep times warrant evaluation by a sleep specialist. Ask yourself what you can change in your life to get the sleep you need. The changes you make might just be life changing.

Michael Jackson

The fact that insomnia has the very real potential to wreak havoc on people's lives is tragically illustrated in the circumstances surrounding Michael Jackson's death. According to the coroner, the pop star died from a lethal dose of propofol, which Jackson reportedly received routinely because of his chronic inability to sleep. However, during the wrongful death trial, Dr. Charles Czeisler opined that Jackson was suffering from total sleep deprivation and that the sixty days of propofol administration rendered Jackson unable to get REM or restorative sleep—leaving him dangerously sleep deprived. Apparently lab rats that are similarly deprived of REM sleep die in five weeks. Dr. Czeisler felt that Jackson's memory loss, chills, paranoia, and a host of other problems could be attributed to sleep deprivation. It is not known why Jackson failed to be treated by a sleep disorder specialist.

CHAPTER TEN

YOU ARE WHAT YOU SLEEP

We are such stuff as dreams are made on;
and our little life is rounded with a sleep.

—William Shakespeare

So you want to be successful, and you think sleep may be an issue? You've come to the right place! In this chapter you'll learn how to get the sleep you need to think like a fully alert person, play the violin like Jascha Heifetz, pole vault like an Olympic athlete, and more.

What we'll show you is that failing to get sufficient sleep leads to multiple levels of cognitive impairment. We'll also prove to you that restoring sleep to optimal levels will reverse these brain deficits.

WHY SLEEP LOSS STUNTS YOUR BRAIN

Sure, *stunts* is a strong term, but we do need compelling language to describe what sleep deprivation is doing to the brain. If you're the type of person who has to close her eyes during the scary parts of horror movies, you may want to turn the lights up before you read the next few paragraphs, because we're going to give you the facts. Those facts don't paint a pretty picture of what happens to the brain when it doesn't get the sleep it so desperately needs.

First of all, sleep-deprived brains become less capable of making moral judgments. Now, here comes the Stephen King–like horror part that we warned you about. In order to understand this brain dysfunction—specifically, how the sleepless brain lacks moral integrity—we need to bring up the peculiar case of Phineas P. Gage, a nineteenth-century railroad worker whose brain was injured when a dynamite blast drove a large iron rod completely through his head (see page 109). The injury destroyed his left eye and much of his left ventromedial prefrontal cortex. Because that region of the brain regulates various aspects of social and emotional reasoning, he experienced a change in his social and moral behavior.[1] As one of his biographers put it, Gage lost the ability to express himself in social situations, and he lost the ability to understand others.[2]

> To act human, you mix emotions, actions, routines, customs, manners, words, and expressions in a predictable way. That's what Gage seems to have lost. Bossing a railroad construction gang requires more than a loud voice. A gang has to be able to "read" the social behavior of the foreman. They have to know if he's angry or just joking, if his orders are reasonable, or if his judgment can be trusted. He has to be able to "read" the social behavior of his men, to know who are the reliable ones and who are the troublemakers. By all reports, the old Gage was an excellent foreman. The new Gage was not. All these changes were brought on by a hole through a specific part of his brain.

When you experience sleep deprivation. you're effectively experiencing the same kind of destruction to your prefrontal cortex that Phineas Gage suffered when the rod passed through his skull, albeit on a lesser level. Unfortunately for Gage, there was no way to repair the physical damage that had been sustained to his cortex. Luckily for you, however, there is a way to repair the damage to your brain's social and moral sense, and that is through obtaining sufficient quality sleep to make up for your sleep debt.[3]

There is no question, however, that sleep deprivation causes this kind of debilitating brain dysfunction, which leads to "low moral awareness the next day."[4] Such dysfunction, which is experienced by all who suffer sleep loss, means that sleepless people are somewhat like zombies. They cannot recognize how other people are feeling, and their unexpressive body language makes it difficult for other people to recognize how *they* are feeling.[5] Their sleep loss puts them in a kind of cocoon where they're isolated from others because they can't recognize social cues, and they're unable to give others the proper social cues to *their* state of mind. Naturally, this type of brain dysfunction is especially problematic when it's incurred by those upon whom we rely for making critical and morally correct judgments, such as judges, police officers, and members of the military.[6]

> Perpetrators of domestic violence typically have high rates of insomnia and snoring, and complain of major sleep loss to their victims.

SLEEP BOOSTS BRAIN FUNCTION

We weren't joking when we said that getting sufficient sleep can help you play the violin like an expert. In a classic study of expertise, K. Anders Ericsson examined the lives of expert violinists and found that of all the activities they did during the day, the two most important were practice (not surprisingly) and sleep. Yes, the best violinists practiced more than the merely good ones, *and they slept more*! This was a key finding, and one that Ericsson emphasized in his report: the best of the best in any field, including athletes and musicians, sleep the most.

More specifically, Ericsson says that of the "eight activities judged to be highly relevant to improvement of violin performance, only two [stand out as having] an average duration ... exceeding 5 hours per week. These two activities were practice alone (19.3 hours per week) and sleep (58.2 hours per week)."[7] He goes on to observe that the best violinists slept 8.6 hours per day, and their teachers slept 7.8 hours per day. The best violinists also took the most naps, averaging 2.8 hours per week. Teachers, in contrast, napped only 0.9 hours per week. Not only do the best violinists sleep more than the merely good ones, they also realize that sleep is vital for their improvement. Ericsson tells us that expert violinists "rated sleep as highly relevant for improvement of violin performance."[8]

> The best violinists sleep 8.6 hours a day and average 2.8 hours of naps per week.

Ericsson also mentions that Olympic athletes sleep for close to eight hours a day, and in addition they take a half-hour nap each day. This serves to boost mental clarity and concentration, two key elements needed for athletic success. Naturally it also boosts physical ability and accelerates tissue repair, as we discussed in Chapter 7.

One of the reasons sleep helps you learn is that during the REM stage people often dream about the tasks they performed earlier in the day. In a recent study, players of the electronic game Tetris were awakened during REM stage sleep and asked what they were dreaming about. "Tetris!" was the usual answer. Those who dreamed about it the most improved their play the most. Researchers said: "Our laboratory has established a direct relationship between the 'replay' of recent experience in dream content, and enhanced memory performance in humans."[9]

The message is clear that you can gain an advantage over your competition—like the best violinists and Tetris players did—by sleeping adequately after performing a task.

SLEEP AND MORAL DECISIONS

Another researcher looking at how sleep impacts who we are is William D. Killgore. Associate professor in the department of psychiatry at McLean Hospital, Harvard Medical School, Dr. Killgore has focused his research on the intriguing area of higher order cognition and executive function. The term *executive function* means the ability of the brain to plan ahead, which involves such skills and abilities as working memory, organization, task flexibility, and carrying out plans.

Dr. Killgore specifically looked at how chronic sleep deprivation impairs brain function. If you are a coffee lover, you'll be glad to know that he has also examined the issue of whether your morning cup of coffee can ameliorate the brain dysfunction that sleep deprivation saddles you with. As we'll see, it cannot.

> I drink coffee because without it I'm basically a two-year-old whose blankie is in the washer.
>
> —ANONYMOUS

Along with other researchers, Dr. Killgore found that sleep deprivation impairs moral capacity. More specifically, it limits our ability to integrate emotion and cognition to guide moral judgments. Along these lines, he found that lack of sleep causes people to take longer to decide upon a course of action when their decision involves a situation that is emotionally charged.[10] It's as if a sleep-deprived brain is operating at a slower speed when dealing with moral issues.

He also discovered that sleep deprivation decreases emotional intelligence. Emotional intelligence is the ability to be aware of the emotions of other people, the ability to use your emotions constructively to get work done, and the ability to manage your own emotions and those of other people by cheering them or calming them as needed. Remember, this was the ability that Phineas Gage lost when the metal rod went through his prefrontal cortex. Dr. Killgore and his associates found that sleep deprivation results in the following negative effects:

- Less assertiveness
- Less impulse control
- Reduced self-confidence
- Less ability to delay gratification
- Reduced empathy for other people
- Greater reliance on superstition and magical thinking

In short, "sleep loss produces temporary changes in cerebral metabolism, cognition, emotion, and behavior consistent with mild prefrontal lobe dysfunction."[11] This is definitely something you want to avoid as much as possible when you're working with other people since it makes it harder to deal with them in a cordial and pleasant way.

As if this loss of emotional intelligence weren't bad enough, it turns out that stimulants—such as coffee and dexies[12]—won't help you get over these brain dysfunctions. *Stimulants may keep you alert and awake, but they can't fix the problems with suboptimal decision making caused by a lack of sleep.* More to the point, sleeplessness leads to poor decision making on tasks that rely on emotion-processing regions of the brain, such as the ventromedial prefrontal cortex, the same area that Phineas Gage lost when the iron rod went through his head. According to Dr. Killgore, "deficits in decision making were not reversed by commonly used stimulant countermeasures, despite restoration of psychomotor vigilance and alertness."[13] It looks like coffee and other stimulants aren't going to solve the problems of sleep loss nearly as well as getting adequate makeup sleep.

The impaired decision making caused by sleep loss can't be restored by coffee or other stimulants; it can be restored only by sufficient makeup sleep.

INCREASING ETHICAL BEHAVIOR

Interestingly enough, there has been a demonstrated association among ethics, deviant behavior, and sleep. Poor sleep quality is related to decreased ethical behavior. Michael Christian of the University of North Carolina's Kenan-Flagler Business School and Aleksander Ellis of the University of Arizona's Eller College of Management studied sleep-deprived nurses and students. Not surprisingly, they found in the sleep-deprived nurses poor performance on tasks requiring strategic planning, risk analysis, and innovative thinking.

What was surprising, though, was that the sleepy subjects displayed deviant and unethical behavior, including rudeness, cheating, and taking more money than they had earned. These findings of increased unethical behavior may be explained by the fact that sleep deprivation acts on areas of the brain that are more primitive than the prefrontal cortex. Besides social and emotional reasoning, the prefrontal cortex controls executive functions, providing skills to make plans, organize, remember things, prioritize, and get started on tasks. These functions help the brain organize and act on information in a rational manner. But by inadvertently promoting sleep deprivation, many industries and organizations are increasing their vulnerability to deviance and unethical behavior.

DON'T GAMBLE ON A SLEEP-DEPRIVED BRAIN

Do you like gambling, playing cards, or taking a calculated risk now and then? Even if you gamble only for fun, the effect of sleep loss on this behavior might interest you. There's nothing wrong with this kind of activity, but don't try it on a night when you're sleep deprived, says Dr. Killgore.

If you gamble when you're tired, you risk losing more money than when you're fully rested. It may sound like common sense, but it's now officially a scientific fact: sleep-deprived gamblers make poor decisions.

Now, while we're at the casino, let's see what the research can tell us about how your date will react when they're sleep deprived. Or, to put it more bluntly, should you date a sleep-deprived man or woman? You might be surprised at what the studies say about this question. Sleep loss apparently affects risk taking and altruism differently depending on gender. This is because sleep deprivation affects the prefrontal cortex, a part of the brain involved in such matters, and because men and women approach risk in different ways and react differently to sleep loss. In a recent study it was found that "sleep deprivation causes a *decrease* of risky choices in females and an *increase* of risky choices in males. Moreover, women become more selfish after sleep loss."[14] So if you're on a date with a sleep-deprived guy, you can expect him to make riskier choices, including when he's driving you home. And if you're on a date with a sleep-deprived woman, you can expect her to be more self-centered and less likely to take a chance on you, to paraphrase the famous Abba song.

Who knew that sleep loss caused such different effects! But knowing these test results will help you in other ways, too, as we shall see shortly.

HOW TO RESTORE BRAIN DYSFUNCTION

Although sleep deprivation is an insidious process and often happens without our being aware of it, if you're like most people, you can sometimes feel the slowness of your sleep-deprived brain, especially when you have lost a lot of sleep in a short period of time. In such cases, you know you aren't your normal jovial self. You realize that other people find you somewhat of a bore, and you also know that you can't read their emotions as well. The $64,000 question, of course, is "What can I do to restore my brain to its bright and optimal functioning level?"

Granted, lack of sleep impairs our prefrontal cortex, just as the prefrontal cortex injury impaired Phineas Gage, but the wonderful thing is that we can fix those problems with sufficient sleep. In fact, good sleep is associated with high positive emotions.[15] Having such a positive mind-set will make it easier to deal with people at work. You'll also enjoy enhanced emotional expressivity and be better able to communicate with others if you get enough sleep.[16] This kind of cheerful disposition is especially important for those who interact on the job with the general public, such as tellers, cashiers, and salespeople. But it's also essential for professionals like accountants, lawyers, and therapists since they want to develop rapport with their clients.

In our opinion, the research in this chapter says something important about how sleep effectively *makes us who we are*. When sleep is good, when we get enough of it, the very act of sleeping strengthens our moral sense, boosts emotional intelligence, and lifts our mood. Put another way, sleep affects us far beyond mere cognitive functioning or physical performance: it contributes measurably to forming our personalities and making us who we are as individuals. The implications of this research are profound, for if sleep impacts intelligence, outlook, disposition, communication, morality, judgment, and confidence—all factors making us *who we are*—then this means that we can take active steps to protect and improve these fundamental components of our lives. By protecting sleep and avoiding the quagmire of sleep deprivation, we can be the best we can be.

Too many people have failed to realize that doing something as simple as obtaining sufficient sleep has the powerful potential to improve who we are, how we see the world, and what we can accomplish with our lives. Sleep fuels optimism, intelligence, rationality, and clarity. And if we can be smarter, happier, and even better people by getting sufficient sleep, we really owe it to ourselves, and to those who we care about, to make the right choice and prioritize this personality-strengthening gift of nature.

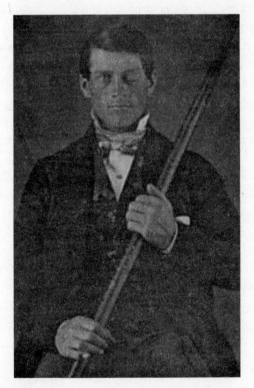

Phineas P. Gage (1823–1860), brain-injury survivor, holding the tamping iron that injured him. Based on original photograph from the collection of Jack and Beverly Wilgus.

Arguing at Bedtime

"Never go to bed mad," said Phyllis Diller. "Stay up and fight."

This humorous advice may contain a kernel of validity, provided, however, that you limit your arguments to *earlier in the day*. Arguing or having serious discussions at bedtime can produce a negative effect on sleep. We see couples that get in bed, turn out the lights, say good night, and then one will say, "I need to talk with you about your son." For many people with busy lives, the only available time for serious discussions might be in those moments prior to sleep. But even if this is the only time when you can secure someone's full attention, it's a terrible time for deep discussions. Try, instead, to schedule upsetting conversations as far from bedtime as possible.

Variations of this theme are reading technical or work-related material until lights out, rehearsing a discussion you want to have with your boss, or reviewing difficult financial circumstances as you're waiting for sleep. It may be easier to agree with a bed partner not to discuss certain topics right before bed than it is to agree with *yourself* not to think about certain things. The room is dark and quiet, and your mind may gravitate toward topics that are inherently distressing. Remember, you have sixteen hours each day in which you can choose to worry. You don't have to spend precious night hours on this activity. Admittedly it's easier said than done, but . . . *let it go*.

David had a patient who finally realized that one aspect of her active mind at night was that she was rehearsing her day so that she would not forget something the following day. She kept a journal on her bedside table and would write down all her thoughts. Once a thought was permanently on that notepad, she could let it go. The next morning she could pick up her journal and begin worrying where she left off.

Some people are so organized and disciplined that they *schedule worry time* during the day. They'll set aside forty-five minutes to do nothing but worry. When the time is up, they let it go with an understanding that they can worry again the following day.

CHAPTER ELEVEN

WHO'S ON TOP?

A light supper, a good night's sleep, and a fine morning have often made a hero of the same man who, by indigestion, a restless night, and a rainy morning would have proved a coward.
—Lord Chesterfield

In 2013 David and I attended a sleep conference in Baltimore. One night we went to dinner with some colleagues, including a relative of the inventor of the water bed. While we were waiting for our food, I happened to glance across the room and noticed a distinguished-looking man sitting with a small group of people. He had white hair and looked very familiar. When I realized who it was, my heart leaped.

"Look, David. Do you see who that is?"

David turned his head. "Sure. It's William Dement. What about it?"

"You can't just sit here so calm like that. You have to introduce me."

"Why?"

"Why! Because Dement is my hero. Come on, let's go. I mean, the man almost single-handedly built the field of sleep medicine. He's done so much, and yet he always manages to protect his own sleep. He's an example of putting your money where your mouth is. This is the opportunity of a lifetime."

David smiled and got to his feet to humor me. By the time we finally arrived at the other table, I had nearly lost the ability to speak. Running through my mind were all Dr. Dement's accomplishments, especially the fact that he had founded the world's first clinical sleep laboratory, at Stanford University. I was reduced to a tongue-tied adolescent and might as well have been meeting the president. I'm embarrassed to admit that I was barely able to utter a hello, but it was still the high point of the conference for me. Dement was very gracious as we interrupted his dinner, and he spent a few minutes chatting with us. To be able to meet the man who had made so many significant discoveries in sleep medicine was really a thrill for me.

I mention this story to make an important point about sleep, one that has the potential to help you in working with other people. You see, Dr. Dement was a real hero to me, a true leader in the field of sleep research. And great leaders evoke positive responses in other people. A wealth of research demonstrates that leaders who get sufficient sleep are more likely to evoke this kind of loyalty and dependability in their followers.[1]

Politicians get on average only 5.1 hours of sleep per night.

POLITICALLY SLEEPING

Bill Clinton was admittedly an insomniac. He enjoyed a reputation for making middle-of-the-night phone calls—basically ignoring his sleep needs and the needs of those around him. Whether or not he had sleep problems prior to becoming president, he candidly and accurately chalked up some of his mistakes as well as some of the edginess of Washington to sleep deprivation. While in office, Mr. Clinton was well known for sleeping only five to six hours per night. Rumor has it that he began to compress this sleep schedule after a professor at Georgetown told him that "great men require less sleep." After leaving office, he described the sleeplessness of politicians:

> But one of the reasons Washington is so . . . you're going to all laugh when I say this, and you're going to think, "He's like everybody else. You know, when they get out of office they get a little dotty and a little crazy." But I'm telling you, one of the reasons that there is often such an acrimonious atmosphere in Washington is that too many members of the Congress in both parties are sleep deprived.

LEADERS NEED EMOTIONAL INTELLIGENCE

One of the most important traits of a good leader is the ability to understand other people. Such understanding involves empathy, the ability to know how others are feeling, and a sense of their level of commitment to your shared goals. It's also important to be able to approach people in a way that makes them glad to work with you rather than annoyed at your lack of sensitivity. Collectively, these people skills are known as emotional intelligence.[2]

Now, wouldn't it be nice if there were some way for you to improve your emotional intelligence? You would get along better with people, and they would enjoy working with you more. With greater emotional intelligence, leading a team would be easier because you would understand the mind set of your employees, and they would be able to read you, too, sensing when you considered something important or when you were just joking with them. Well, research reveals that you *can* improve your ability in all these areas by getting sufficient sleep.

The reality is, we're not paid by the hour as leaders. We're paid for creativity and innovation. It's not about the amount of hours; it's about
the passion and enthusiasm and quality of our ideas. And that quality
is directly impacted by how we take care of ourselves.

—DAN CATHY, businessman

This means we can look forward to getting along better with people
when we're well rested. The prefrontal cortex, remember, is that part of
the brain that Phineas Gage lost when a metal rod penetrated his skull.
As a result of that accident, he lost the ability to be an effective railroad
foreman since he could no longer read other people, and he was so bland
and expressionless that no one could read him, either.[3]

LEADERS COMMUNICATE WELL

By all accounts, Ernest Shackleton was a soft-spoken man. Regarded as
one of the most effective leaders of all time,[4] he is known to have kept
his cool even under circumstances that would have made an ordinary
man quail. When ice crushed and sank the ship that brought him and
twenty-seven men to Antarctica, stranding them thousands of miles
from civilization, he is reported to have said, "Boys, now we go home."
This type of calm communication motivated the sailors to have courage
and do what was necessary to preserve their lives.

You can achieve similar heights of communicative excellence
provided you obtain sufficient sleep. If leaders were well rested, a recent
white paper on leadership contends, "They would be functioning at
their best, with better memories and stronger skills for making new and
creative connections. They could regulate emotions and more effectively
engage with others. Stress would decrease. The complexity of leading
would be matched by the capability to respond with clarity, creativity,

and productivity."[5] Fail to get that sleep, and you risk major rifts with your followers. General Patton, for example, had difficulty sleeping during the Allied invasion of Sicily in World War II,[6] and he slapped two soldiers. Hardly a way to enhance communication. It was a breach of discipline that resulted in both the press and his superior, General Eisenhower, rebuking him.

All effective leaders need a way to recharge their batteries so that they can communicate better. Sleep is undoubtedly the most effective method to accomplish this recharging. One of the ways that sleep improves your ability to communicate is that it actually makes your face physically brighter and more expressive. A recent study demonstrated that sleep measurably affects features of the eyes, mouth, and skin. It perks up the face and fosters better communication between people.[7] Sleep also elevates our mood[8] and makes it easier for us to relate to our employees in a positive manner. It's no wonder that sleep should be a leader's best friend.

Many leaders find it relaxing to read before bedtime. General Patton was known for using this strategy. His favorite reading material was Field Marshall Erwin Rommel's book on infantry tactics.[9] Not exactly light reading, but to each his own.

LEADERS NEED GOOD JUDGMENT

Leaders have an ethical obligation to use good judgment.[10] This is nowhere more important than in politics and the military, where poor judgment could result in bad legislation or even substantial civilian casualties.[11] In a study of the need for sleep and the effects of sleep deprivation on behavior and performance in the military, it was discovered that sleep functions to optimize soldiers for combat effectiveness. According to the study, "As sleep debt accumulates, a person's mood, motivation, attention, alertness, short-term memory, ability to complete routines, task performance . . . and physical performance will become . . . negatively affected."[12] All these negatives impair the exercise of good judgment by military personnel.

The converse is also true: sufficient sleep is associated with better judgment. Soldiers returning from Iraq as part of Operation Iraqi Freedom who got adequate sleep experienced less depression, less post-traumatic stress disorder, less panic, and less need for reliance on tobacco and alcohol. They also made fewer attempts at suicide.[13] The implications for the military are obvious: sleep management strategies need to be implemented so that soldiers in combat situations can obtain more sleep.

The wider implication for managers in the civilian world is equally clear: only by obtaining sufficient sleep can leaders be assured of maintaining the mental equilibrium needed to exercise good judgment. In fact, by obtaining sufficient sleep, leaders preserve thalamic gray matter, which is used in decision making. The thalamus relays sensory information from the outside world to the appropriate areas of the brain for processing. Without a functioning thalamus, it is difficult to make good decisions. In fact, high thalamic activity has been detected in decision making in male adolescents.[14] Managers who obtain sufficient sleep can expect to preserve this important brain area, allowing them to make better decisions.[15]

> Long-term total sleep deprivation reduces thalamic gray matter volume in healthy men.
>
> —CHUNLEI LIU, sleep researcher

CLEVER LEADERS ARE GOOD LEADERS

One of the chief characteristics of Odysseus, the king of Ithaca and the hero of Homer's epic poem *The Odyssey*, is his cleverness. Homer calls him "resourceful" many times throughout the narrative. Although the hero of the poem is a creature of Homer's imagination, his reputation as a crafty and thoughtful leader is known the world over. Indeed, cleverness is a good quality for a leader to have, for by being thoughtful and creative you can show your followers useful new ways to do things, just as Ernest Shackleton, for example, coached his men in new ways of surviving on the ice.

It should come as no surprise that sleep can help you develop the resourcefulness needed to lead successful enterprises. Studies show that REM stage dreaming enables the brain to consolidate memories and put sensory data together in creative new ways.[16] A recent study highlighted this helpful feature of sleep. "It has become clear that the sleeping brain offers an ideal environment for solidifying newly learned information in the brain," the authors concluded. "Sleep . . . supports the consolidation of many different types of information. It not only promotes learning and memory stabilization, but also memory reorganization that can lead to various forms of insightful behavior."[17]

One of the researchers involved in this study, Jessica Payne, a cognitive neuroscientist at the University of Notre Dame, put it this way: "The sleeping brain isn't stupid—it doesn't just consolidate everything you put into it, but calculates what to remember and what to forget."[18] Yes, sometimes even more important than the ability to remember is the ability to forget. By allowing the mind to let go of the flotsam and jetsam of the day, sleep helps put the spotlight on what is truly important.

LEADERS VALUE SLEEP

Good leaders value sleep. Calvin Coolidge slept eight hours a night, plus two or three hours in the afternoon. In fact, his very first act as president of the United States was to go to sleep. It is said that Calvin Coolidge got more sleep in the White House than any other president.

"No matter what time it is, wake me, even if it's in the middle of a Cabinet meeting," said Ronald Reagan.

George W. Bush made sure that he usually got to bed on time and was rested for the next day's work. This strategy allowed him to maintain a level of competence during the political and military crises that occurred while he was president, including directing the Afghanistan and Iraq invasions.

"Every important mistake I've made in my life," Bill Clinton said, "I've made because I was too tired." His outspokenness and frankness reflect a mature understanding of the value of sleep for a leader. If more leaders got more sleep, the world might be a safer place for us all.

In 1916 Ernest Shackleton and five British sailors undertook the most daring open-boat voyage in history, traveling eight hundred miles in sixteen days across the stormy Drake Passage in the southern Atlantic Ocean. The trip was so perilous that they almost froze to death, and they were severely sleep deprived. When they arrived at King Haakon Bay on South Georgia Island, Shackleton knew his men were close to the breaking point. The cold and lack of sleep during their voyage had sapped them of all strength. So he found an ice cave and ushered them into it. He took a double watch, allowing his navigator to sleep. This was his reward for Frank Worsley, the man who had charted the lifesaving course for the little boat using just a compass and sextant.

Unfortunately, during their harrowing two-year adventure there was not much time for sleep on the ice floes and in the small rescue boats after their ship was crushed by the ice and sank, stranding them far from home. But Shackleton ordered his men to sleep when they could, revitalizing their morale and stamina. This was one of the strategies which enabled him to do the near impossible and bring them all home alive.

The great explorer's action illustrates an important lesson: *exceptional leaders ensure that their people get sufficient sleep.* The fact that a good leader encourages *others* to sleep is also emphasized by a white paper issued by the Center for Creative Leadership.[19] It recommends that leaders establish employee sleep programs at their places of employment. The purpose of such programs is to teach people the value of sufficient sleep. If you're a manager, part of your success will depend on having employees who are sufficiently rested to do their job well. So taking this advice to heart is bound to lead to greater success in your organization, just as it helped Shackleton bring all his men home after two years on the ice.

PART THREE

ALL YOU NEED IS SLEEP

CHAPTER TWELVE

GET A ROOM

The bed has become a place of luxury to me! I would not
exchange it for all the thrones in the world.

—Napoleon Bonaparte

"I can't sleep, Terry."

"Can you describe your bedroom?"

"Better yet, I'll show you a photo."

I was in my office talking with a thirty-four-year-old photographer.
She had taken some very nice wide-angle shots of her bedroom. She
held her laptop up for me to see.

When I saw the photos, my heart sank. I had seen this problem
before. Many times, in fact.

"I'm pretty sure I know what the difficulty is," I said.

"But how's that possible?"

"Just from looking at these photographs."

Her sleeping area was a shambles. The small bed was unmade, heaped
high with sheets, pillows, clothes, and towels. Stacks of photographs and
a broken tripod leaned against the wall. Shoes and boots peeked out
from beneath the bed. A basket of laundry was beside the door and . . .

"A jumbled setting is typical of a lot of creative people," I said.[1] "But
research tells us that it's definitely not conducive to sleeping well. So I'm

not surprised that you're experiencing a problem with your sleep. You're young and in good health, so I suggest you try some tips about the bedroom that I'd like to share with you today. I don't see why they wouldn't help you get a better night's sleep."

"What would you like me to do?"

I outlined the following tips and tricks for how to arrange the sleeping area. As you'll see, some of these ideas are similar to sleep hygiene rules in chapter 18, but they all specifically apply to giving your bedroom a makeover. The purpose is to rearrange the space so that it resembles the most serene, relaxing, and visually appealing bedroom you've ever seen.

THE VALUE OF ORDER

In the quest for a good night's sleep, the importance of having a therapeutic sleeping environment can't be overstated. For all intents and purposes, your bedroom should be considered a sleep sanctuary. It must be designed with a single purpose in mind, namely to provide a peaceful, inviting, comforting setting, one that is highly conducive to relaxation and sleep. A secondary goal can also be to make it look alluring for intimacy with a partner.

The ancient Chinese developed an effective system of harmonizing architectural spaces. Called feng shui, it requires that the bedroom be your ultimate inner sanctum. For example, all closet and bathroom doors leading into the sleeping area should be closed when you turn in for the night. There should be ample space on either side of the bed. Something beautiful and inspiring should be placed where you will see it upon awakening. This ancient method of interior design, which is practiced by many modern architects, also requires that you avoid using the space under the bed as a storage area.

Some of the principles of feng shui appear to have a basis in scientific fact. Keeping the bedroom tidy and clutter-free, for instance, generally promotes better sleep. A minimalist décor prevents the mind from becoming distracted by clutter. Disorder can produce stress, and according to the American Psychological Association, stress is the number-one cause of short-term sleep problems such as frequent middle-of-the-night waking and insomnia. Paperwork, bills, unfolded laundry, unfinished projects, and exercise equipment should all be moved out of the bedroom. In this way, the bedroom will be associated more strongly with only sleep and intimacy.

BEDDING

What happens when you go to a five-star hotel? Your room has a bed with fresh linens. Sometimes there's even turndown service, where a staff member enters the room and turns down the bed linen for you, leaving a mint on top of the pillow. Several surveys have demonstrated that most people prefer crawling into a well-made bed with freshly scented sheets at night. It's the kind of luxurious experience that can promote feelings of well-being and a greater sense of relaxation. The takeaway point here is that a neat and organized environment improves mood and reduces stress.[2] It may be worthwhile to keep your bed neat to see whether that makes bedtime more pleasurable and relaxing, as well as making your sleeping environment more aesthetically appealing. These factors alone may serve to contribute to an improved night of sleep.

TEMPERATURE

Keep your bedroom dark, quiet, and on the cool side. The ideal temperature is between sixty-eight and seventy-two degrees. Some researchers have recommended wearing socks and even gloves to bed if needed. A study at the sleep laboratory in Basel, Switzerland, discovered that wearing socks in bed can increase the chances of falling asleep. Swiss researchers found that when the feet and hands are warm, blood vessels dilate, allowing heat to escape and body temperature to fall, initiating sleep. Conversely, when hands and feet are cold, the vessels constrict, retaining heat, which may keep you awake. Cold feet can also serve to interfere with the release of melatonin.[3]

You can buy mattresses and mattress pads that will heat or cool the sleep surface. Some of these are dual zoned for bed partners with contrasting temperature preferences. Many people find that the temperature of the sleep surface is more closely associated with comfort and sleep quality than the room temperature. Sleep-surface temperature manipulation can help with sleep latency (the time it takes to fall asleep) as well as sleep maintenance and waking. Manipulating the temperature of the sleep surface may be more sleep inducing than piling on extra blankets, and it may also be more cost effective than excessively heating or cooling the bedroom. Let's not forget to mention that individualized sleep-surface temperature manipulation may help foster better relationships.

> The good news is, there's more and more awareness about the power of a good night's sleep. [But] what we're doing in America is, we're drugging people to make it through the night on, in many cases, a lousy bed.
>
> —DAVID PERRY, executive editor, *Furniture/Today*

LIGHTING

Starting two to three hours before bedtime, dim the lights in your home. Lowering the lights signals your brain to produce melatonin, the hormone that brings on sleep. Use a 15-watt bulb when reading in the last hour before bed. Installing dimmer switches in your bedroom can be helpful in lowering the light levels prior to sleep.

Be aware that there may be numerous sources of sleep-disrupting light in your sleeping environment. Digital clocks, DVRs, cell phones, and laptops need to be covered or removed.[4] The blue wavelengths of light emitted by these devices interfere with sleep. Turn off all electronics an hour before bedtime. Cover any displays you can't shut off. We know of a super sleeper (a person who takes sleep seriously) who designed his house so that he can shut off all electricity in the bedroom at night, allowing for zero possibility of ambient lighting from any source.

While it's a good idea to use blackout drapery to block light from outside, especially if you live in the city, these curtains don't have to be heavy or dark in color. Lighter-colored curtains and appealing fabrics in a variety of textures can block light effectively, provided that they're lined with blackout material. Layering visually appealing blinds, sheers, and drapes, all of which can effectively reduce light, is also an option.

Some people recommend positioning your bed to the east in order to wake up seeing the sun's rays. If that's not practical, upon arising go to the sunniest room or venture outside and expose yourself to sunlight for fifteen minutes. In the daytime, try to get as much exposure to natural light as possible. This will stimulate your body's sleep-wake mechanism and aid in your transition into sleep at night.

NOISE

Few people realize that noise can be as detrimental to quality slumber as a sleep disorder. This is because noise can wake you up several times throughout the night, just like sleep apnea, without your even realizing it.

The sleeping brain registers and processes sound. Unlike the visual system, the auditory system continues to monitor the environment and will arouse the sleeper in response to a potential threat. This built-in safety mechanism is why an unfamiliar noise will wake you more so than a familiar one. Different people have different tolerances for noise, but on average a sound above fifty-five decibels (such as a ringing telephone) will cause you to awaken. However, even if a noise doesn't fully wake you up, it can produce other disturbances. For example, it can cause an increase in your heart rate and blood pressure, changes in breathing, and restless body movements. These physiological effects occur with sound exposure levels as low as forty decibels (such as a loud whisper). Some intriguing new research indicates that if you can lower the noise level in your bedroom by a mere 5.8 decibels, you can expect to measurably increase the quality of your sleep.[5]

Noise in the bedroom tends to fragment sleep, which in turn will suppress immune function. This negative effect occurs even if you don't wake up.

For people who don't like earplugs, white noise machines that mimic rainfall, ocean waves, or other natural sounds can be installed. Or you can just let your exhaust fan or air conditioner lull you to sleep. Even though these white noise sounds may be loud, they work by distracting the brain and making it pay less attention to other sounds that might otherwise wake you up.

> I don't care what women say, size matters in bed. The bigger the bed,
> the more room you have to move around.
>
> —NIKHIL SALUJA

MATTRESSES

Professor Chris Idzikowski, director of the Sleep Assessment and Advisory Service in Edinburgh, found that people with uncomfortable mattresses experience an average sleep loss of one hour per night. But let the buyer beware: the selection process of a mattress is a very personal matter. It's hard to believe that many people purchase one without even trying it. Which brings up the next point: mattress comfort is wildly subjective. One person's dream bed is another person's nightmare. This is due to the many variables that individually constitute comfort. In short, don't count on the fact that your bed partner will like the mattress that you find most comfortable.

Mattresses need to be supportive enough to keep the body properly aligned while sleeping, and comfortable enough to be relaxing. A good mattress should be large enough for you and your bed partner to move around on easily. Although the queen is the most popular bed size in America, a king-size mattress will provide extra room and may be well worth the investment if it results in better sleep quality.

Another factor to think about when considering a mattress is that as we age, skin becomes less elastic, increasing sensitivity at pressure points. This means that a mattress with more padding will feel more comfortable. Many people find that the mattress that felt comfortable in their thirties is not right in their sixties.

SEX AND THE MATTRESS

When you think about beds, two things probably come to mind: sleep and sex. It's a good idea to consider *both* when mattress shopping. A mattress that leads to good sleep doesn't necessarily lead to good sex. For instance, the popularity of foam mattresses over the last few years has led to mixed reviews when it comes to sex. Foam has been criticized for providing a tractionless surface and has also been described as "like having sex in quicksand." One irate reviewer in Miriam Gottfried's 2012 "Sleep or Sex?" Barron's report said, "It's like shagging on a ball of clay." Another mattress reviewer's complaint about foam consisted of "losing a pretty good rhythm" while on it.

If discretion is a concern, it's obvious that you'll want to avoid an innerspring mattress since it produces more "bounce" and noise than foam. A foam mattress has the advantage of being much quieter and is unlikely to telegraph what's happening to your neighbors.

Latex and innersprings enjoy high ratings for ease of movement, according to a Sleep Like the Dead survey. Air beds, in contrast, were criticized for the partition in some models as well as their noisiness. In our final analysis, after considering all the options and weighing the various pros and cons, we suggest choosing a mattress for better sleep, not better sex, since better sleep ultimately leads to better sex.

Sleep Positions

As soon as infants are able to roll over independently, sleep position preferences begin to form. By age seven most children have established a preferred sleep position. It's estimated that the typical adult changes position from three to thirty-six times per night. Excessive position changes are related to poor sleep quality, with good sleepers changing sleep positions less often than poor sleepers.

INCOMPATIBLE BEDFELLOWS

If you think *you* have problems getting comfortable with your bed partner, just consider that in *Moby Dick* Ishmael has to share a bed with a tomahawk-carrying cannibal. As the story goes, they finally make it through the night and become good friends. Your problems can't be nearly as difficult, but it's certainly true that having an incompatible bed partner can interfere with good sleep.

When it comes to bedroom temperature, some like it hot, some like it cold. Some prefer lots of blankets and pillows; others prefer a minimalist approach. Some people toss and turn, bothering their partner and waking them repeatedly. Snoring is also a big, disruptive problem for the partner who must listen to it. Sleeping together or apart may mean the difference between sleep deprivation and quality sleep.

In ancient Rome the marital bed existed for one purpose and one purpose alone, and that didn't involve sleep. Before the Victorian era, it was the norm for married couples to sleep apart. The concept of bed partners is a fairly recent one, and it only came about as a result of cramped quarters and restricted living space in overcrowded cities. While Lucy and Ricky, Rob and Laura, and a host of other TV characters kept separate beds for the sake of censors, sleeping together has been seen in modern times as a culturally accepted indicator of being in a committed relationship—but it may or may not be a prerequisite to healthy, restorative sleep.

While many couples enjoy sleeping together, others find that the sleep interruptions caused by their bed partner negatively impact their night. Such interruptions can even cause relationship problems. Since most of us slept alone throughout our childhood, the sudden transition to sharing a bed with a partner can prove comforting for some and problematic for others. This transition to sharing a bed can lead to either sufficient or inadequate sleep, depending on the individual circumstances. In any event, you may be amused to learn that even the researchers are not in bed together on this one: they appear to be completely polarized on the topic.

> I blame my mother for my poor sex life. All she told me was "The man goes on top and the woman underneath." For three years my husband and I slept in bunk beds.
>
> —JOAN RIVERS, comedian

APART

Contrary to popular belief, sleeping apart and good relationships are not mutually exclusive. Sharing a bed is certainly not conducive to good sleep for some couples. In fact, many loving, happy, and committed couples report sleeping apart in order to get undisturbed, quality sleep that can actually be beneficial to a relationship. The National Association of Home Builders has even seen an increase in homes with two master bedrooms, with 60 percent of all custom upscale homes now having two owner suites.

Most polls and surveys on sleeping together or apart estimate that up to a quarter of cohabitating couples choose to sleep separately due to the fact that they sleep better without a bedfellow. A 2012 survey by the Better Sleep Council found that 26 percent of respondents reported sleeping better alone. Bed partners should consider sleeping apart if one or both lose sleep as a result of sleeping in the same bed. While convincing research indicates that married couples are happier and healthier than singles, the advantages of living together can be compromised by disrupted and fragmented sleep resulting from sharing a bed.

For couples who share a bed, one partner's sleeping problem can easily become a problem for both. It's not unusual for the one who is unable to sleep to harbor resentment toward the partner who is able to get shut-eye. One British survey found that cosleeping problems caused 75 percent of respondents to consider leaving their partners. Many of our patients come to see us only because their bed partner has moved out of the bedroom or is threatening to do so if something is not done to correct the snoring.

> Contrary to popular belief, sleeping apart and good relationships are
> not mutually exclusive.

Snoring is the single most commonly cited reason for sleeping in separate beds. The Better Sleep Council's 2012 survey found that partner snoring and tossing and turning keeps women up at night more than men. Snoring has been documented at close to ninety decibels, which is the equivalent of a motorcycle revving its engine. Oddly enough, snorers are oblivious to the noise and, if awakened, will deny that they were snoring. Obviously a bed partner's sleep is improved when the snorer is treated. It is important to note that snorers should always have sleep apnea ruled out.

Yet it's not only snorers that can cause problems; other constant disturbances can be just as debilitating. Neil Stanley, a sleep researcher at the University of Surrey, firmly believes that the secret to a long and happy marriage is sleeping in separate beds. In one study, Stanley found that couples who shared a bed suffered 50 percent more sleep disturbances. It has been demonstrated that when one partner moves during sleep, there is a 50 percent chance that the other will change position in response to the movement. This can add up to excessive position changes and poor sleep quality. Reasoning that poor sleep increases the risk of stroke, depression, car accidents, heart disease, and divorce, Stanley advocates the ancient Roman approach as the key to a happy relationship: bed sharing for sex, not for sleep.

TOGETHER

While Stanley and others maintain that disrupted and shortened sleep resulting from bed sharing can be harmful to your health and relationship, proponents of cosleeping cite research that emphasizes the health benefits of bed sharing. Paul C. Rosenblatt, professor emeritus at the University of Minnesota, interviewed forty-two couples ranging in age from twenty-one to seventy-seven for his book *Two in a Bed: The Social*

System of Couple Bed Sharing. Rosenblatt concluded that the upside of cosleeping includes better health, a better sex life, and an increased sense of security. He emphasized that people have to learn how to share a bed and that the benefits of physical and emotional intimacy outweigh the negative aspects of bed sharing.

Researchers including Dr. Wendy Troxel at the University of Pittsburgh believe sleeping next to someone helps lower the stress hormone cortisol, possibly because it promotes feelings of safety and security. Cosleeping may even lower levels of harmful proteins called cytokines, which are associated with inflammation, autoimmune disorders, heart disease, and depression. Bed sharing can also boost levels of oxytocin, the love hormone, which is known to promote bonding. Originally believed to be released only during sex, its production may also be associated with cuddling in bed.

In a study published in 2009, Troxel found that women in long-term stable relationships fell asleep more quickly and woke up less often during the night than women without a partner. She concluded that the stable presence of a bed partner promotes better sleep quality in women.

Proponents of bed sharing note that bedfellows have the distinct advantage of being able to detect health conditions in each other, such as sleep apnea, seizures, and diabetic shock. Keep in mind that sleeping in separate beds rather than seeking medical attention for conditions such as snoring, kicking, and sleepwalking can be dangerous to your physical health and is never recommended. If cosleeping leads to better sleep, then by all means arrange to do it. If not, don't be afraid to try sleeping apart to see if your sleep quality might improve.

WHOOPEE

Sleep affects numerous aspects of our lives, including sex. As with many other aspects of our functioning, a bidirectional association exists between sleep and sex. Years ago, prominent sex researcher Alfred Kinsey noted that the basic lifestyle factors of sleep, diet, and exercise are important to our sex lives. Not surprisingly, researchers have found lower libidos and less interest in sex in both men and women who are sleep deprived. A 2009 Consumer Reports survey of one thousand adults reported that the top reason couples gave for avoiding sex was "too tired or need sleep." For many people, sexual activity serves to improve sleep, so it may be worthwhile to rest up and conduct some of your own "sleep research."

It may also be that sleep plays a role in the more complex dynamics of a relationship. Amie Gordon, a psychologist at the University of California, Berkeley, analyzed heterosexual couples and found that people tend to feel less grateful toward a romantic partner if either they or their partner generally sleeps poorly. Gordon concluded that poor sleep negatively influences relationships, affecting emotions related to gratitude and appreciation. Interventions directed at improving either quality of sleep or relationships may provide overall benefits, as the two directly impact one another.

So, what happened when our photographer patient tried these suggestions? She was highly motivated, and not only did she manage to do many—though not all—of the techniques, she also brought me several eight-by-ten glossy photos of the result. I have them on my office wall to this day. She was beaming as she told me her response.

"My bedroom is soothing now."

"And how is your sleep?"

"I look forward to going to bed. I sleep much better and more soundly. I'm less distracted and have fewer worries when I turn in for the night. In the daytime I have more energy. My clients seem very happy with me, and I'm doing more work than ever . . . There's only one drawback."

"What's that?"

"Everything is so neat, I keep feeling that I'm in a hotel. I'm constantly wondering why there's no room service."

We had a laugh over her little joke, but the results of our experiment were clearly positive. Getting rid of the clutter in her bedroom worked wonders. In truth, her sleeping space is a model of appropriateness now. It looks like something you might see in *Architectural Digest*: rather minimalist and, most importantly, tidy. It's no wonder she sleeps more soundly. And it's no surprise that she's more successful with her business.

Bedroom Blues

Blue bedrooms apparently lead to peaceful sleep more so than bedrooms of other colors, according to some interior decorators. Sleep experts speculate that the good results in blue rooms may be due to the fact that the color blue is associated psychologically with calmness. In fact, a survey conducted by Travelodge.co.uk found that the color blue also reduced blood pressure and heart rate, two factors that can contribute to restful sleep.

The second most effective color, according to the survey, was yellow. Green and silver came in third and fourth as sleep-promoting colors. The bedroom colors that caused people to have the most difficulty falling asleep included purple, brown, and gray.

CHAPTER THIRTEEN

SLEEP ENVY

The worst thing in the world is to try to sleep and not to.
—F. Scott Fitzgerald

We recently saw a young man from west Texas. He was working for an oil company. He was sent to see us because he fell asleep while driving and ran into the only tree in the county.

People with sleep disorders can sometimes experience dangerous transitions from being awake to falling asleep. This is why it's so important to treat these disorders. Without doubt, the most common sleep disorder is insomnia. The word "insomnia" is a broad term implying insufficient sleep or poor sleep quality. It's estimated that as many as sixty million Americans occasionally experience insomnia. They're unable to sleep on a regular basis. That means that in any given year, about a third of the population will have some difficulty sleeping.

When sleep clinicians talk about insomnia, they use a slightly more precise definition of the word. If you keep our definition in mind, you'll be talking like a sleep expert. Our definition focuses on the individual's problem sleeping and on the consequences of that problem for daytime activity. So when we talk about insomnia, we mean an inability to get sufficient sleep, together with some form of daytime impairment.

After we explain in more detail what insomnia is, and what causes it, we'll tell you about the most effective methods of treating it. You can be assured that this sleep disorder can be treated successfully.

WHAT IS INSOMNIA?

The term *insomnia* first appeared in 1623, originating from the Latin *in* (meaning "not") and *somnus* (meaning "sleep"). However, this is a misnomer for most people who complain about insomnia. That is, most people with insomnia don't complain of *no* sleep; rather they complain about getting too little sleep, having difficulty falling asleep, waking frequently during the night, or waking too early and being unable to return to sleep. Some people even complain about nonrestorative sleep (sleeping but getting little benefit from the sleep). The same individual may experience any or all of these symptoms, and symptoms may vary from night to night. To be classified as insomnia, sleep difficulties must also be associated with at least one of the following daytime problems.

- Fatigue or malaise
- Daytime sleepiness
- Mood disturbance or irritability
- Concerns or worries about sleep
- Impairment in concentration, memory, or attention
- Workplace or driving accidents or errors
- Academic, social, or vocational dysfunction
- Reduced motivation, energy, or initiative
- Headaches, GI symptoms

The inclusion of daytime symptoms helps differentiate insomniacs from natural short sleepers.

WHAT CAUSES INSOMNIA?

We once saw a woman in her fifties who reported severe difficulty falling asleep. When we inquired about her bedtime routine, she said that she would get drowsy on the couch, would get up to brush her teeth, and then would put on her nightgown. She would get in bed and be unable to fall asleep. When we asked for more details, we found that she had conveniently left out one important aspect of the routine. On further inquiry she reported, "I brush my teeth, brush my hair, put on my nightgown, call my mother, turn out the lights, and I cannot fall asleep." The phone call to her mother was a curious omission, and when asked about it, she admitted that her mother despised the man that our patient had married. Her mother would spend thirty minutes berating the man and emphasizing how disappointed she was that her daughter had married him. This occurred almost every night. When she hung up, the woman was so upset and angry that any hope of quickly going to sleep was lost. We asked her to stop calling her mother, but she said she would feel guilty and that would hinder sleep. So we made a compromise: she could call her mother first thing in the morning, not at night. Her day was shot to hell, but her nighttime sleep improved.

This story illustrates one of the interesting facts about insomnia: there can be any number of different causes. Age, gender, health, and mental conditions are the strongest factors associated with the disorder. Older age is associated with increased insomnia, but this may not be due to age per se but rather to increased medical problems, medications, sedentary lifestyle, and decreased social activities. Women are twice as likely as men to report insomnia complaints. Health and emotional conditions can increase the incidence of insomnia substantially compared with individuals without these conditions.

Insomniacs Charlotte and Emily Brontë reportedly would walk in circles around the dining room table until they got sleepy.

Insomnia complaints can be classified as transient, acute, or chronic. Transient insomnia lasts for several days. If poor sleep lasts several weeks, it is classified as acute insomnia. Chronic insomnia may last for one month to several years and can wax and wane in severity over that time. Studies indicate that chronic insomnia affects 9 to 17 percent of the American population.

Most acute insomnias can be traced to a trigger or cause. For example, sleep may worsen as final exams approach, or a major business deal is being negotiated. Once the exams are finished or the deal is closed, sleep generally returns. The trigger for chronic insomnia is usually lost to history, and many people report that their sleep began to gradually worsen over a period of time without any clear reason why. However, some people can identify a period of stress, such as going through a divorce or the loss of a loved one, which started the problem.

There are a number of physical and psychological factors that increase the risk of insomnia:

- Stress
- Medication use, side effects, and discontinuation
- Lifestyle factors (poor sleep habits, excessive caffeine use)
- Environmental conditions (noise, extreme temperatures)
- Circadian system disruptions (jet lag, shift work)
- Mental health disorders (depression, substance abuse)
- Neurological disorders (Parkinson's, Alzheimer's)
- Other sleep disorders (apnea, restless legs syndrome)
- Medical disorders (hyperthyroidism, cardiovascular conditions, joint and low back pain)

In its initial stages, insomnia occurs when predisposing factors, such as the tendancy to be a worrier, combine with precipitating or triggering factors, such as life stress, to create problems with falling asleep, midnocturnal or early morning awakening, or diminished sleep quality.

Once insomnia begins, perpetuating factors, including ineffective compensatory behaviors (e.g., daytime naps, sleeping in on weekends, going to bed earlier to get rest) and negative thoughts (*I will never fall asleep*), create a vicious cycle, transforming an acute problem into a more chronic one. Without an intervention, the ineffective coping strategies distort an individual's sleep-wake cycle, while the negative sleep thoughts trigger anxiety and create a self-fulfilling prophecy: *If I believe I can't fall asleep, then it's likely that I'll be tense at bedtime and find it difficult to sleep.*

Primary insomnia. The term *primary insomnia* implies that poor sleep need not be caused by emotional or health factors but can occur on its own in a person free of significant depression, anxiety, or medical illness. The most common primary insomnia is called persistent psychophysiological insomnia. We also call it a learned insomnia. The theoretical cause of this type of insomnia is a combination of somatized tension with learned sleep-preventing behaviors.[1] "Somatized tension" means that stress is expressed through physiological channels (muscle tension, increased heart rate) rather than cognitive channels (overt worry). The learned sleep-preventing behaviors include a marked preoccupation with sleep. This may be a natural response to not sleeping. For example, if your car is working properly, you rarely think of it during the day; however, if the battery is failing, you may think of little else. The same is true with sleep. When we're sleeping well, we take it for granted. When we're not sleeping, as bedtime approaches we can't help but dread the coming struggle.

> Some thoughts are too angry to sleep. They lie awake all night and become obsessions.
>
> —MARTY RUBIN, author

Obsessing about sleep will lead to an attempt to try to sleep. This is usually a mistake since "try" is an arousing word. Instead, sleep must be allowed; it has to overtake you. It can't be forced. The more you try to sleep, the more agitated you'll get that it's not happening. This agitation will lead to more arousal, and a vicious cycle is in place. People with this type of insomnia often find that they fall asleep at times when they're not trying to do so. They may fall asleep on the couch watching television or while reading a fascinating book about sleep.

We also know that sleep can be conditioned. Some people have a specific position in bed that means they're serious about sleep. For example, some may lie on their back once they get into bed, and think about their day or what to expect tomorrow. When they're ready for sleep, they turn to their stomach, raise the right arm, crook the left leg, and "assume the position" that has always been associated with falling asleep. It turns out that people who have made an association with a specific body position and falling asleep in fact fall asleep more quickly than those who have never made such an association.

Likewise, not sleeping can also be conditioned. If you've spent night after night struggling to sleep, the bed, the bedroom, and even your bedtime ritual can become associated with poor sleep. Individuals with this form of conditioned insomnia may notice that they, too, can fall asleep on the couch, but once they get up and begin the bedtime routine, they feel less sleepy. By the time they get into bed, they're wide awake. Some people with this type of insomnia will sleep better in locations other than their bedroom. They sleep better in hotels or at a friend's home. They sleep better on the couch or in a guest room. We even see that these people, to their embarrassment, sleep better in the sleep lab than they do at home. They sleep better outside their own bedroom because these other locations haven't been conditioned with poor sleep.

TREATING INSOMNIA

Sometimes treating insomnia requires a clinician to understand a person's entire life story. For example, we saw a college senior who developed a severe insomnia during her last year at college. She was expected to graduate on time, but as graduation approached her sleep problems got worse. Her history revealed that she was from a wealthy family and, upon her graduation, her father was planning to buy her a business to run. She was personally not interested in running a business and did not feel that she was ready for such a responsibility. But as long as she had a severe sleep problem, her father agreed that she could not run a business. This was a combination of stress over an anticipated event and secondary gain: provided that she was sick, she could avoid an unpleasant situation. Treatment in this case involved helping this young woman deal with a demanding father in a more direct manner.

People who wish to treat their insomnia are sometimes surprised when they find out the details of some of our most effective approaches. For example, it seems natural to people to spend more time in bed when they're sleeping little; however, this is one of the worst things that you can do. Many people will go to bed earlier to "try" to get more sleep. They may stay in bed longer hoping to prolong their sleep. They may spend more time in bed for "rest" even though they're not sleeping. While at first glance increasing time in bed seems to be the correct response, with a little information you'll see why this is the wrong approach.

> Van Gogh poured camphor on his mattress and pillow in an attempt to alleviate his insomnia. The treatment may have led to his mental problems and suicide.

If your body is happy getting seven hours of sleep (anyone with sleep problems would probably be very happy to get seven hours of continuous sleep), and you decide to spend nine hours in bed to try to get that sleep, you have just guaranteed two hours of wakefulness. Even if you have been having many nights of poor sleep, your body may not get more than seven hours on a good night. With a seven-hour sleep need and nine hours in bed, you will be awake for two hours sometime during the night. It may take you two hours to fall asleep, or you may wake up early and find it impossible to get back to sleep. More likely, you'll start to sleep in bits and pieces, getting a few minutes or hours of sleep interspersed with periods of wakefulness. Seven hours of sleep in one block is much better than seven hours of sleep spread out over nine to ten hours.

There are other reasons spending more time in bed isn't a good response to poor sleep. With a guarantee of two hours of wakefulness, your mind will have more time to wander and gravitate to problems. You'll also be associating the bed and bedroom with wakefulness, causing a conditioned response to poor sleep. Finally, since circadian rhythms are alerting in the early evening, if you go to bed too early, you'll back into the "forbidden zone," where sleep is very difficult even if you are sleep deprived. This is an important point. Even if you take a medication during the alerting portion of your circadian cycle, the medication is apt to be less effective than if you wait until these alerting rhythms are diminished. The same medication is likely to be a great deal more effective if taken one to two hours later.

WHAT'S SO SPECIAL ABOUT INSOMNIA?

When treating insomnia, the first place to start is with sleep hygiene. *Good sleep hygiene is important for all sleepers, but particularly for those with insomnia* (see Chapter 18). Still, we need to stress here that treating insomnia is very different from treating other sleep problems. Throughout this book we have emphasized things such as the importance of getting more sleep, spending more time in bed, and adhering to schedules. With insomnia, at first glance it appears that we'll be contradicting ourselves. More often than not we recommend that people spend less time in bed, pay less attention to their sleep, and delay their bedtimes.

The ideas we're discussing about the importance of sleep are just as true for the insomnia patient. *However, in order to improve sleep, we sometimes have to gain more control over the process of sleep.* We can usually gain this control by employing systematic sleep deprivation and by decreasing the preoccupation with sleep that might otherwise lead to arousal.

The point is that many sleep hygiene rules have to be approached differently for the insomniac. For instance, for normal sleepers (that is, noninsomniac sleepers), the main issue is taking sleep seriously. This includes prioritizing sleep, going to bed at a regular time, and increasing total sleep time. For insomnia patients, however, the issue is almost the opposite: they need to take sleep *less* seriously and not adhere to a rigid schedule. Insomniacs need to realize that they can function on less sleep and, if anything, at least temporarily decrease total sleep time so that sleep quality, time to fall to sleep, and number of awakenings can be improved. In other words, general advice to all sleepers does not necessarily apply to the insomniac; insomnia patients are different. Advice that would be good for normal sleepers is actually counter to what we recommend for insomniacs. We don't think this approach is a huge issue, but it needs to be thought through because you can get painted into a corner. For example, naps are good, unless you have insomnia; going to bed at the same time each night is good, unless you have insomnia; and spending more time in bed is good, unless you have insomnia.

SLEEP RESTRICTION THERAPY

With an understanding of the role of homeostasis and circadian rhythms in controlling the timing and duration of sleep (see "The Two Factors of Sleep Control" on page 19), treatments can be designed to take advantage of both these factors and improve overall sleep quality. Alcohol is one of the few substances that increases stage 3 NREM sleep. However, it is well known that sleep deprivation also increases this sleep stage.

Stage 3 NREM is very deep sleep, difficult to awaken out of, and perceived as good-quality sleep. One way to improve this sleep stage is with a treatment called "sleep restriction therapy." It's important to understand the theory behind this before simply undertaking it. We have many patients who say they will do anything to get their sleep back. However, once we start talking about sleep restriction therapy, they almost immediately say, "Well, I'm not going to do *that*." Initially, sleep restriction therapy seems counterintuitive. If one is not sleeping, why curtail sleep time even more? But once we explain the rationale, most people are willing to make the effort.

FAMOUS INSOMNIACS

Marilyn Monroe
Alexandre Dumas
Michael Jackson
William Shakespeare
Napoleon Bonaparte
Franz Kafka
Abraham Lincoln
Madonna
Margaret Thatcher
Judy Garland
Sir Isaac Newton
Emily Brontë

The important point about sleep restriction therapy is that it's a controlled form of sleep deprivation. The key word here is "controlled." By determining how much sleep you get most nights, you can set a baseline to begin the therapy. For example, if you typically get five hours of sleep most nights, with sleep restriction therapy you're limited to only five hours in bed. We generally feel that the wake time is more important than the bedtime, so we typically will set a wake time and move backward from there. If you absolutely need to be out of bed by seven in the morning, then bedtime becomes 2:00 a.m. You have to get up at

7:00 a.m. whether or not you slept. We also prohibit napping during the day. Once sleep begins to improve, we gradually move your bedtime earlier. Once you get three consecutive nights with 90 percent of the time in bed asleep, you go to bed fifteen minutes earlier. Stay at this bedtime until you achieve another three days with 90 percent of the time in bed asleep, then move your bedtime fifteen minutes earlier. In a gradual manner, sleep time increases and bedtime becomes earlier.

This technique takes advantage of both homeostasis and circadian rhythms. We tend to delay bedtime, which puts us well past the forbidden zone and on the falling leg of the temperature curve. By limiting the time in bed, we increase the homeostatic sleep drive with a consistent, though modest, sleep deprivation. With this technique, you can begin to fall asleep more quickly and awaken less often during the night. Awakenings become shorter in duration. One caveat: this technique doesn't work immediately, and there may be no benefit for several days after beginning treatment. As a result, you need to commit to trying this approach for a few weeks before deciding whether or not it's effective.

Michael Jackson died trying to sleep. One of the drugs that killed him, benzodiazepine, is prescribed for insomnia.

LIGHT THERAPY

Some insomnias based on a circadian rhythm disturbance are amenable to light manipulation. This treatment uses a combination of behavioral therapy and bright light. We typically put a light box on a bedside table with a timer that comes on forty-five minutes before the person needs to be out of bed. These lights can radiate up to 10,000 lux. A typical office light is only about 320 to 500 lux. So 10,000 lux may sound blinding, but in fact it's the equivalent of morning sunlight and is actually quite pleasant. This exact same light is used to treat seasonal affective disorder

(SAD). However, with the circadian rhythm disturbance, it's not the light per se but the timing that makes the difference. Morning bright light can help you fall asleep earlier in the evening. Evening bright light does just the opposite: it causes you to stay up later and sleep later the following morning. So, for example, for teens who like to stay up late and sleep late, morning bright light will help them fall asleep earlier and wake up better in the morning. Unless they put their head under a pillow, the light will produce a phase-advancing effect. For older people who have difficulty staying awake in the early evening but who wake up at 4:00 a.m. and can't return to sleep, bright light in the evening can keep them awake longer and help them sleep later. Considering the powerful effect that light can exert on circadian rhythms, it's no wonder that sleep clinicians are so concerned with how people are exposed to light before, during, and after sleep.

STIMULUS CONTROL THERAPY

Another technique for treating insomnia, developed by sleep researcher Richard Bootzin, is called "stimulus control therapy." The idea behind this approach is a concept we discussed earlier, that is, both sleep and wakefulness can be conditioned or associated with your environment. When you have spent many nights staring at the ceiling and waiting for sleep, the bed and bedroom can be conditioned to stimulate poor sleep. Bootzin reasoned that this conditioning could be changed so that the bed and bedroom could, once again, be a signal for good sleep. He developed a technique designed to reassociate the bed and bedroom with sleep instead of wakefulness. To do this, people are coached to go to bed only when they're sleepy, not just because it happens to be 10:00 p.m. If they haven't fallen asleep in about fifteen minutes, they are instructed to get out of bed and engage in some relaxing behavior, such as reading, until they're once again sleepy. Only then should they return to bed. This step is repeated until the person is able to fall asleep within fifteen minutes of retiring. The rationale for this form of conditioning is that the bed will be limited to sleep and sex. We want the bed to have a strong stimulus effect for sleep.

The stimulus value of an object is based on ideas demonstrated by Pavlov's dogs. Pavlov was able to show that he could elicit salivation in a dog by sounding a tone that was always paired with food. After a short period of time, the tone alone would elicit salivation even if no food was present. The tone had become a stimulus to eating and this elicited the salivation. Now, please don't get insulted that we're comparing sleep patients to Pavlov's dogs. Our point is simply that the stimulus control approach really has value. What Bootzin is trying to do is pair your bed with sleep so strongly that the bed itself will elicit sleep for you.

CONTROLLING THOUGHTS

Virtually everyone with a sleep problem has a dialogue going through their mind about the cause and consequence of poor sleep. In fact, most of us have a dialogue going through our minds continuously, assessing all aspects of our lives. While it is usually in the background and often unnoticed, it is possible to start listening to this dialogue and to challenge some of the content. For example, many people have a tendency to catastrophize. That is, they tend to imagine the worst possible consequence and take that consequence at face value. We recently saw a gentleman who had a very good job and, in fact, his wife also had a very good job. He was not sleeping well, and his internal dialogue revealed that he truly believed that if his sleep problem was not solved, his whole family would be homeless and living under a bridge. The thought process was: *I need to provide for my family. If I can't sleep well, my performance will be impaired. If my performance is impaired, I won't be able to do my job. If I can't do my job, I'll lose my business. If I lose my business, we'll have no money and I'll go into serious debt. We'll then lose the house and be living under a bridge.* The poor fellow was almost completely unaware of this dialogue until we had him listen to what he was telling himself.

Although becoming homeless is a theoretical consequence of poor sleep, it's extremely unlikely. Other common examples of inner dialogue might include, for example, a feeling that if I don't sleep well tonight, my day will be ruined, I'll have a nervous breakdown, or I'll get sick and need to be hospitalized. While each of these might be a possible consequence of poor sleep, each would, again, be extremely unlikely. If you start hearing this dialogue and questioning it, there's a good likelihood that you can limit the negative effects these thoughts have on your sleep. For example, the man who thought his sleep problem would lead to homelessness began to question the belief by noting that he had never been homeless, was actually making a good living, and even if he did lose his job, his wife could easily support the family. By questioning the unrealistic belief about being homeless, he was able to put more accurate cognitions in place, and doing so took a great deal of power away from the insomnia.

Guided Imagery

An active mind at bedtime is common, and in fact an active mind can serve people well under most circumstances—except at bedtime. If your mind is active at night, try to use this to your advantage: work *with* your strengths. That is, engage the mind in some manner that allows sleep rather than hinders it. For example, use an active mind to visualize yourself in a pleasant environment. Mentally picture yourself on a sunny beach and use as many of your senses as you can. Feel the sun against your skin and the wind in your hair. Hear the surf hitting the pebbles and the sound of a distant gull. Smell the salt in the air. This creative use of the imagination can be profoundly relaxing, and at the same time it has the added advantage of *focusing cognition and preventing worry from intruding into your thoughts*. The visualization distracts you from the fact that you're in bed and not sleeping, and it may allow sleep to overtake you.

COGNITIVE BEHAVIORAL THERAPY

During cognitive behavioral therapy (CBT), you're taught to pinpoint false notions that may interfere with sleep. For example, you may think you need eight hours of sleep when your body can actually get by on seven. You're also taught to deal with negative thoughts or concerns that might keep you awake at night and to change certain behaviors, such as caffeine consumption. CBT typically includes between four and eight hour-long sessions led by a sleep therapist, and may also include meditation, muscle relaxation, biofeedback, or hypnosis.

In essence, CBT is a psychotherapeutic method used to teach people how to recognize and change patterns of thought and behavior to solve their problems. CBT specifically for insomnia treatment is referred to as CBT-I. The goal of CBT-I is to break a person's negative thought process and anxiety over sleep. CBT-I is a practical approach, emphasizing good sleep hygiene, a bedroom environment conducive to sleep, getting in bed when sleepy, and getting out of bed when unable to sleep. It is short term and goal oriented. In the past decade, this type of therapy has emerged as an exceptionally effective treatment for insomnia.

> CBT is one of the few treatments that has shown any lasting progress
> in the successful treatment of insomnia, typically providing relief to
> 70 to 80 percent of people who use it.

In one study, researchers concluded that cognitive behavioral therapy is more effective and lasts longer than a widely used sleeping pill, zolpidem, in reducing insomnia. Sixty-three otherwise healthy people with insomnia were randomly assigned to receive cognitive behavior therapy, zolpidem, both, or a placebo. Study subjects in the CBT group received five thirty-minute sessions over six weeks. They were given daily exercises to "recognize, challenge, and change stress-inducing" thoughts, and they were taught to delay bedtime or get up to read if they were unable to fall asleep after twenty minutes. The patients taking zolpidem were on a full dose for a month and then were weaned off the drug. At three weeks, 44 percent of participants receiving cognitive therapy and those receiving combination therapy and pills fell asleep faster compared with 29 percent of patients taking only sleeping pills. Two weeks after all the treatment was over, all patients who had received CBT fell asleep in half the time it took before the study, while only 17 percent of patients taking sleeping pills fell asleep in half the time.[2]

In fact, CBT-I is one of the few approaches that has shown any lasting progress in the successful handling of insomnia, typically providing relief to 70 to 80 percent of those who have completed treatment.[3]

CREATIVITY AND INSOMNIA

Recent research has supported a theory of creative insomnia, in which creativity is significantly correlated with sleep disturbance. In a 2010 paper, D. Healey and M.A. Runco explored a possible link between creativity and insomnia in a study of thirty highly creative children and thirty control children, hypothesizing that there would be a higher rate of sleep disturbance in the creative children. Results confirmed that creative children did have more sleep disturbance than noncreative children, suggesting that creative ability may affect sleep patterns. Oscar-nominated actor George Clooney, for example, was open about the fact that he had problems with insomnia. Yet he admitted that he did some of his most successful screenwriting during bouts of sleeplessness. Honoré de Balzac, the French novelist, was also known for doing his best work in the wee hours of the morning. These and other stories about successful people raise the intriguing question: Is insomnia sometimes the result of ambition and creativity?

It is important to maintain reasonable expectations about sleep. The lifetime incidence of insomnia is 100 percent. What this means is that everyone occasionally has difficulty sleeping. If you've had difficulty sleeping and begin to improve, a bad night might well throw you off track again with a mistaken belief that a poor night means chronic insomnia is returning. In reality, you need to expect that you're going to have an occasional bad night. A particularly stressful day, an argument with your spouse, a difficult project at school, or trouble at work can certainly cause a temporary disruption in sleep. Keep in mind that one bad night doesn't mean that the chronic problem is returning. It simply means you're normal.

Problems in the Middle of the Night

I can tell you with some certainty that no matter what problem you have ever had in your life, it is tenfold worse at three o'clock in the morning. If you're dwelling on problems at three o'clock, they'll *seem* catastrophic and unsolvable, and you may feel hopeless. If you can just wait until 10:00 a.m., the problem may not go away, but it will be much more manageable. The reason for this appears to be a basic shift in our brain chemistry and the utilization of different brain circuits to deal with problems during the night. The brain is more emotional during the night, so even small problems seem huge. No matter what solution you come up with at three in the morning, you're going to have to rethink it when your brain is working in a more logical manner. I know it may be difficult, but if you find yourself grappling with that catastrophic problem in the middle of the night, tell yourself to let it go. Have faith that the problem will be less daunting if you allow your brain time to become more logical and less emotional. You're not going to have a good solution to that problem at 3:00 a.m., and you'll need to rethink it later. It's destroying your sleep. Let it go.

CHAPTER FOURTEEN

GOOD IN BED

Ignorance about sleep is the worst sleep disorder of them all.

—William Dement, *The Promise of Sleep*

You might find it hard to believe, but sleep research can be fun. Maybe a little story by David will illustrate what he's talking about. My mentor, Howard Roffwarg, worked with William Dement in New York. As we have mentioned, Dement is the father of sleep medicine. Well, Dement would perform sleep studies in his Manhattan apartment back in the day, just like Freud, who analyzed patients in his living room. Only Dement took it one step further. He usually conducted his studies on Rockettes. While the dancers were sleeping, Roffwarg would station himself in the bathroom of the apartment to analyze the recordings.

There's no question that my friend and colleague Andrew Jamieson had a good sense of humor about his job. He was the first fellow at the Stanford Sleep Center, and he worked closely with both Dr. Dement and Christian Guilleminault, another pioneer in sleep research. Dr. Guilleminault coined the terms *obstructive sleep apnea* and *hypopnea* and has published more than six hundred articles in peer-reviewed medical journals over the years. Whenever Jamieson and I had an idea for new research, Jamieson would remember his days at Stanford and, with a pronounced French accent to mimic his former teacher, would say, "But Daveeed, we have already done zees study."

I mention these incidents because I think it's good for you to have an idea of what it's like to work as a sleep researcher. It's also important to have a positive attitude, and being able to laugh at yourself is always helpful. I mean, even we sleep researchers don't take ourselves too seriously. Every year there's a national meeting of sleep experts to discuss the latest scientific discoveries on sleep and to share our thoughts. You may find it reassuring to know that not even the experts get it right all the time. As I was riding an elevator with a colleague at one such meeting, he turned to me and said, "Think how many sleep hygiene rules we've broken today." True, that's probably about as wild as this group gets. But it still reflects the kind of upbeat attitude that can help you make progress with your own sleep issues. The point is, you want to focus on your problems, not obsess over them.

Even good sleepers encounter problems every now and then. Some sleep disorders are serious enough to interfere with normal physical, mental, and emotional functioning. Sometimes these disorders can even be life threatening. The Institute of Medicine estimates that between 50 and 70 million Americans suffer from insufficient and poor-quality sleep on a chronic basis. Our best guess is that more than half of these people are experiencing sleep disorders.

The first continuing medical education conference on sleep disorders was held at Stanford University on November 29, 1972. At the time, there were only three known sleep disorders: narcolepsy, restless legs syndrome, and the newly discovered obstructive sleep apnea. William Dement believed that a medical discipline "can only be said to exist if it represents an organized body of knowledge, and if this body of knowledge can be effectively taught." We now recognize and treat more than eighty different sleep disorders. Here we discuss the three original disorders: sleep apnea, restless legs syndrome, and narcolepsy.

Good sleepers report that they get in bed, think about their day or fantasize a bit, and the next thing they know, the sun is shining and it's time to get up. This is the goal we have for you, too: a peaceful night of slumber, what Shakespeare calls the "chief nourisher in life's feast."[1]

Sleep Disorder, Anyone?

A positive response to two or more of these questions could indicate sleep deprivation or a sleep disorder.

- Are you often cranky and irritable?
- Do you have trouble thinking at work?
- Are you experiencing a lot of stress?
- Do you move frequently during sleep?
- Do you nod off during the day?
- Have you had trouble falling asleep or staying asleep for a month or more?
- Do you react slowly?
- Do you have high blood pressure?
- Do you snore?
- Are you told by others that you look tired?
- Do you sleep for eight hours yet still feel tired?
- Do you experience problems falling asleep or falling back asleep?
- Are you overweight?
- Are you sleepy during the day?
- Do you have a large neck size?
- Do you have to take a nap every day?
- Do you wake up with morning headaches?
- Do you find it hard to stay awake while driving, watching TV, reading a book, or attending a meeting?

SLEEP APNEA

"I don't have sleep apnea."

"How do you know?"

"I've never had the problem."

I was talking with a forty-seven-year-old accountant who had just been tested in the sleep lab. He had experienced episodes of impaired breathing more than two hundred times during the night. And yet the amazing thing was that he had no knowledge of the fact.

"Are you sure you don't have it?"

"Well, Doc, I would know, wouldn't I?"

"No, not necessarily."

"What did my test results say?"

I broke the news to him about the hundreds of times he had difficulty breathing during the night.

"But—but—how could that be right? I mean, how could it have happened to me so many times and I have no memory of it? I think your test must be wrong."

"The answer is very simple. These arousals to breathe are very brief, only a few seconds. You then immediately return to sleep before your consciousness has recorded the event. But look at the results yourself."

I handed him the test printout. Like many patients, he found it difficult to believe until he saw the results. Fortunately, the disorder is very treatable today, and we have an extremely high success rate.

I explained to the accountant that sleep apnea is a breathing disorder that occurs only during sleep.[2] The word "apnea" comes from Greek *apnoia*, meaning "breathless." Sleep apnea was first described in the medical literature in 1965; however, historical descriptions go back to the nineteenth century. When we fall asleep, the muscles in the body begin to relax. This relaxation also affects the throat muscles. As these muscles relax, they can begin to vibrate, causing a snore. If you make the sounds of snoring, you'll feel that the back of your throat is vibrating. If there's enough tissue in the throat, or if the airway is small enough, the muscles can relax to the point where they occlude the airway completely. The affected person is still trying to breathe, but the tissue in the throat acts like a cork in a bottle. Air can't get through. As a result, oxygen in the blood decreases and carbon dioxide rises. At some point, the brain will awaken to get more oxygen. There is typically a short three- to five-second arousal during which muscle tone returns, the airway opens, and breathing resumes, often associated with a snort or gasp. With the improved airflow, blood oxygen rises and carbon dioxide falls. The brain can quickly return to sleep, usually without sleepers being aware that they awakened. Once they are asleep again, the whole process starts over. This pattern can happen literally hundreds of times during the night, and the sleeper may be completely unaware that it is occurring.

Ironically, the bed partner is usually very aware that breathing is impaired. In many ways it is the worst of all worlds for that bed partner. They are first attempting to sleep in the presence of loud, crescendo-type snoring. These episodes are followed by periods of silence during which it can be obvious that the sleeper is trying to breathe but is unable to get air. Bed partners will vacillate between thinking *I wish he would stop snoring* to *I wish he would start breathing!*

There is a variation of sleep apnea that is in many ways more dangerous because it's less obvious and people may be less likely to seek treatment. In some cases, the airway relaxes but not to the point of complete occlusion. Air is still moving. There are no pauses in breathing, usually just continuous snoring. However, the sleeper is not getting enough oxygen and the same pattern unfolds: periods of insufficient airflow resulting in a drop in blood oxygen saturation and an increase in carbon dioxide, then brief arousals followed by a resumption of normal breathing. These breathing abnormalities are called hypopneas (*hypo* meaning "little" and *apnea*, "not breathing"), and they can be just as dangerous as full obstructive apnea.

The severity of sleep apnea can vary considerably. We look primarily at two factors to determine how serious the problem is: (1) the number of episodes of impaired breathing per hour (called the "apnea/hypopnea index," or AHI), and (2) the blood oxygen level. A higher AHI generally means a more severe problem. However, a low AHI that is associated with severe drops in oxygen level can also represent a threat to health. For adults, we consider a normal level of apnea (that is, not problematic) to be an AHI less than five episodes per hour, with blood oxygen saturations remaining above 90 percent. Severe apnea can produce an AHI reaching forty times per hour or even higher. Blood oxygen saturation in severe apnea can fall to the 50 percent range. This level of oxygen saturation is not compatible with life. Only the arousal and return of normal breathing keeps apnea patients alive.

Men are more likely to develop apnea than premenopausal women, and the condition is more common in Hispanic and African-American men. However, after menopause, women are as likely as men to develop the disorder. This finding suggests that female hormones may protect against sleep apnea. However, using hormone replacement therapy does not predictably improve breathing during sleep. In addition to the effects of gender and age, several other factors can make sleep apnea worse.

Sleeping in the supine position. Sleeping on your back can worsen apnea, primarily because gravity lets the tongue fall straight back, which can narrow the airway. In addition, this position permits the stomach to push up against the diaphragm, making it more difficult to breathe.

Stage REM sleep. During this sleep stage we're paralyzed, and as a result muscle tone in the upper airway is at a minimum. Breathing problems during sleep are usually worse in this sleep stage, and some people have apnea only in REM sleep.

Obesity. The heavier you are, particularly around the neck, the more likely you'll have apnea. The internal lumen, or opening, of the airway can decrease (a bad thing) with weight gain and can increase (a good thing) with weight loss. If you have apnea, gaining weight can make the condition more severe. Weight loss can lessen the severity and in some cases eliminate the problem. About 70 percent of apnea patients are overweight and about 25 percent of overweight adults have apnea.

High altitude. Sleeping at a high altitude can worsen apnea because less oxygen is available and blood oxygen levels can decrease to a greater degree.

Alcohol, muscle relaxants, sedatives, and opioids. Alcohol selectively decreases muscle tone in the upper airway. As a result, some people do not snore unless they have consumed alcohol. Others may snore all the time but don't have apnea unless they have consumed alcohol. Alcohol also decreases the ability to wake up from sleep, which terminates an apnea event. So the duration of an apnea event can increase when alcohol has been consumed.[3]

Physical exertion. Following a strenuous day, snoring and apnea may be worse due to increased relaxation of the upper airway muscles.

Smoking. Here's yet another reason to quit: smoking is associated with significantly increased risk of obstructive sleep apnea.[4] This effect may be caused by the way that smoke alters sleep architecture, upper airway function and inflammation, and arousal mechanisms.[5]

A study published in the *Journal of Clinical Endocrinology and Metabolism* in 2002 suggests that many men with sleep apnea also have low testosterone levels. In the study, nearly half of the men who suffered from severe sleep apnea were also found to have abnormally low levels of testosterone at night.[6] This finding suggests that treating apnea may help increase testosterone to normal levels.

SYMPTOMS OF SLEEP APNEA

It is worth repeating that most people who have sleep apnea don't know it. So it's especially useful to become familiar with the signs and symptoms of this condition so that you can recognize it in yourself and in others. Here's a list of the major symptoms and risk factors for apnea.

Snoring. This is the symptom that alerts most people to seek treatment. However, snoring need not be loud or persistent throughout the night. It's also important to note that many more people snore than have sleep apnea, so although this symptom alone is a sign that apnea might be present, it's not in itself a confirmation of the condition.

Observed pauses in breathing. This is also a good indicator of sleep apnea, but the pattern and frequency of the pauses help determine how significant the problem really is. Normal adults can have some apnea during the night. An AHI of less than five per hour is considered normal.

Daytime sleepiness. This is probably the most common complaint of individuals with sleep apnea. Episodes of obstructed breathing during sleep are terminated by brief and usually unremembered arousals. These episodes disrupt sleep continuity and quality and can cause significant daytime sleepiness, even after a sufficient number of hours of sleep. There is some thought that changes in blood oxygen saturation may also contribute to daytime sleepiness.

Nocturia. Frequent urination at night (at least two trips to the bathroom) can be a sign of sleep apnea. When we breathe against a closed airway, our heart produces a substance called atrial natriuretic peptide (ANP). This is a normal response to an abnormal situation. ANP is a potent diuretic and can increase urination during the night.

Gastroesophageal reflux. Frequent reflux is commonly associated with sleep apnea. The cause is unknown, but some sleep experts theorize that the increased pressure changes resulting from apnea lead to reflux, while others feel that preexisting reflux can trigger apnea.

Changes in attention, concentration, and mood. Sleep apnea can increase the likelihood of depression and anxiety. It can make it more difficult to concentrate, and it may negatively affect memory. These changes may be due to the sleep disruption or blood oxygen changes associated with the disorder.

Dry mouth. Sleeping with an open mouth can be a sign of nasal congestion. Humans prefer to breathe through their nose if they can. But the mouth will open if there's not enough airflow through the nose. An open mouth during sleep will change the mechanics of the support muscles for the upper airway and may put them at a mechanical disadvantage.

Morning headache. Headaches that resolve with wakefulness (that is, which go away shortly after you wake up) and which don't require treatment can be a sign of sleep apnea. They may be caused by changes in blood oxygen saturation during sleep.

Frequent awakenings. Although the large majority of arousals due to apnea aren't remembered, some arousals may lead to full awakenings during the night. An arousal pattern that is fairly consistent (for example, a person who says, "I wake up every one to two hours during the night") could be a sign of a REM-related apnea. REM sleep occurs in ninety-minute cycles, and sleep apnea is typically worse during that sleep stage.

Waking up gasping or choking for air, or feeling as if you were not breathing. While not a common complaint, this is a symptom of concern.

Hypertension. Transient changes in blood oxygen saturation during the night, which are associated with sleep apnea, can also cause changes in blood pressure while the person is sleeping. These disturbances could lead to a change in the set point of the individual's normal blood pressure. Hypertension is common in sleep apnea, and sometimes treating apnea reduces or eliminates the need for medication to control blood pressure.

Neck circumference, and more. A large neck size (seventeen inches or greater in men, sixteen inches or greater in women) is a risk factor for sleep apnea. Having large tonsils, a large tongue, or a small jawbone are also risk factors. There is also evidence of a family tendency to develop sleep apnea.[7]

> Obstructive sleep apnea and other breathing-related sleep problems
> are fairly simple to diagnose and treat, but recognition of the problem
> needs to come first.
>
> —ED GRANDI, former executive director
> of the American Sleep Apnea Association

TREATING SLEEP APNEA

Our ability to treat sleep apnea has improved markedly over the years. Initially, the only treatment that we had available was to perform a tracheotomy, the surgical construction of a respiratory opening in the trachea. This procedure allows the movement of air to bypass the upper airway, which consists of the nasal passages, tongue, and throat. When David began his career, almost everyone in his waiting room had a tracheotomy. If you think it is difficult to get someone to have a sleep study now, it was much more difficult then. But don't worry, tracheotomy isn't considered as a primary treatment today. Modern treatments for sleep apnea include oral appliances, surgery to remove tissue from the throat or to move the jaw forward,[8] weight loss, and positive airway pressure (PAP) devices. Currently, PAP is the most utilized and effective treatment method.

If you're experiencing symptoms that suggest you may have apnea, particularly daytime sleepiness, we encourage you to seek assessment from a qualified sleep professional. Daytime sleepiness can be a very dangerous symptom. The one place that any sleep disorder can be a terminal illness is in your car.

When I woke up this morning my girlfriend asked me, "Did you sleep well?" I said, "No, I made a few mistakes."

—STEVEN WRIGHT, comedian

Assessment. If you're suspected of having apnea, the most likely recommendation will be to have a sleep study. Most people are apprehensive about such a test, but they're completely painless and actually quite easy to undergo. Keep in mind that we want you to sleep. Every effort will be made to make you relaxed and comfortable. These studies are typically conducted in home-like environments with private rooms and amenities such as comfortable beds, televisions, and Internet access. Electrodes are pasted to the head. Then other sensors are placed on the body to measure airflow, breathing effort, heart rhythm, and blood oxygen saturation. These are all noninvasive and don't hurt. The sleep center will try to get you to bed as close to your normal bedtime as feasible. They'll also wake you in the morning to remove the equipment. You're free to go home once the equipment is removed. If you need to use the bathroom during the study, it's quick and easy to get out of bed. Your sleep specialist or physician will then use the results of the sleep study to help determine your diagnosis and treatment options.

Home testing. More recently, many home-testing devices have become available for the assessment of obstructed breathing during sleep. Typically, you'll obtain the device from your sleep specialist or physician. They'll show you how to apply the equipment. You sleep with the device at home and return it after one or two nights of use. A sleep professional downloads and reviews the data. While patients generally prefer these devices since they can be used at home, they typically provide far less data than an in-lab study. For example, most of these devices provide data only on breathing and oxygen saturation. They usually don't provide any data on sleep. This type of test is currently helpful only in diagnosing sleep apnea. It is unable to diagnose other sleep disorders.

A variety of treatment options are available depending on the severity of the disorder. We've been successfully treating apnea in our clinics for many years, and the following are some of the most effective approaches.

1. **Avoiding the supine position.** Some people have sleep apnea only when they sleep on their back. One of the earliest treatments was to sew tennis balls into the back of a pajama top. The idea was that if you got onto your back, it was so uncomfortable that you would immediately turn over. But with this treatment we were just robbing Peter to pay Paul. That is, if the apnea didn't awaken you, the tennis balls would. A more effective technique is to use a body pillow propped up against your back to keep you on your side. There are also commercially available devices, such as pillows and cushions, to help you avoid the supine position. Some people find they can avoid apnea if they sleep on their back with their head elevated.

2. **Weight loss.** As noted earlier, there's a strong relationship between being overweight and having sleep apnea. Moderate weight loss has been shown to eliminate apnea in some individuals. Admittedly, weight loss is difficult under even the best of circumstances, and with even mild sleep apnea you're a long way from ideal circumstances. First, apnea makes you sleepy, and when you're sleepy you're less likely to exercise. Second, sleepy people often eat as a means of staying alert. Third, apnea can affect two hormones, leptin and ghrelin, both of which are important for appetite and metabolism. Apnea alters the secretion of these hormones in a manner that makes it very difficult to lose weight. In many instances, weight loss is more realistically achievable after sleep disorders are addressed and treated.

3. **Dental appliances.** There are dental appliances that work by moving the lower jaw forward. When you use these devices, the space at the back of the tongue is increased. This approach is especially helpful for dealing with snoring and for mild to moderate apnea. The devices are typically made by dentists, and the newer appliances are adjustable. That is, if you're still snoring after being fitted for an appliance, it's possible to move the jaw forward even more to eliminate the snores.

4. **Nasal PAP.** Most people are aware of "the machine" to treat sleep apnea, and some have already decided that they want no part of it. Yet the majority of people find that they feel infinitely better using PAP. The acronym stands for "positive airway pressure." It's a fairly small machine, about the size of a lunch box. The box is hooked up to a mask that covers the nose, or sometimes both nose and mouth. The machine blows air from the room (not oxygen). The air pressure is used to "splint" (support or brace) the upper airway during sleep so that it can't collapse. In our experience, this machine works remarkably well. The whole point of PAP isn't to torture you but rather to help you sleep. And when you sleep, you feel better. Intuitively, it seems that it would be difficult to sleep with a mask on your face. But the reality is that most people do quite well with the device. There are now various types of PAP.[9] CPAP is the most commonly used device and it operates on a set pressure throughout the night. BiPAP has two pressure settings, a higher one when you breathe in and a lower one when you breathe out. APAP is an auto-set device that adjusts the pressure during the night as pressure needs may change. For example, if a higher pressure is needed when

you are supine, this machine can increase the pressure when you move to your back and lower the pressure when you sleep on your side. A nice feature of the machines is that they're very quiet, and you can probably understand that bed partners much prefer a PAP machine's gentle whirr to the sounds of snoring. We also put humidifiers on the machine to limit nasal drying due to the constant airflow. The machines are so small and portable that you can easily travel with them. While it may be a bit of a nuisance to use them, these devices can immediately eliminate even severe apnea in most patients while restoring sleep quality. It's a real understatement to say that the many significant benefits of eliminating sleep apnea far outweigh the machine's slight inconvenience.

We have had a considerable number of patients who experienced such improved sleep after a night of PAP treatment in the sleep lab that they did not want to leave in the morning without a PAP machine in hand. Sometimes, however, patients hate the machine after the first night but come to realize they feel so much better the next day that they decide to try it. A good night's sleep after years of untreated sleep apnea can be a life-changing event.

5. **Surgery.** There are also surgical options for treating sleep apnea. Some of these procedures are under general anesthesia in a hospital, and others may be under local anesthesia in an office. The advantage of surgery is that it can be curative, as it was for Red Sox first baseman Mike Napoli, whereas position monitors, dental appliances, and PAP therapy are treatments. That is, if you don't use the device, you'll still have apnea. The downside of surgery is

that it can be painful in the neck area for a few days or
weeks following the procedure. Surgical procedures are not
always successful, or the apnea may return after a few years.
If you're interested in surgical options, you should see an
otolaryngologist (ENT) to assess your suitability for this
type of treatment.

With an incidence similar to asthma and diabetes, sleep apnea affects
at least 20 million Americans, and yet more than 75 percent remain
undiagnosed and untreated. Estimates of the annual economic cost of
moderate to severe sleep apnea in the United States are $65 to $165
billion. The annual health care costs for people with OSA are two times
greater than for those without.

It stands to reason that sleep apnea is unhealthy. Not only does it
disrupt sleep, leaving people feeling sleepy and exhausted, but if left
untreated, it can cause high blood pressure, sexual dysfunction, stroke,
depression, headache, diabetes, memory problems, weight gain, heart
failure, irregular heart rhythms, heart attacks, and worsening ADHD.
Not to mention that untreated sleep apnea may be responsible for accidents, mood disorders, poor performance, job impairment, academic
underachievement, and motor vehicle crashes—as with any condition
that impairs and interrupts sleep.

A sobering new study from the Mayo Clinic indicates that people with untreated sleep apnea are more likely than those without the
disorder to die suddenly from a heart rhythm problem during sleep.[10]
With this in mind, it's worth noting that sleep apnea is a remarkably
common problem, and it's also very treatable. If you think you may
have sleep apnea, don't hesitate to discuss it with your doctor. The good
news is that accident and health risks return to normal after people are
diagnosed and treated for sleep apnea. Unfortunately, apnea was determined to be a contributing factor to Reggie White's untimely death at
age forty-three, just four years after ending his football career with the

Carolina Panthers. With size putting him at risk for the disorder, the thirteen-time Pro Bowler's weight often topped 290 pounds. Research has shown that sleep apnea is unusually common among NFL linemen due to their size, as weight is a major factor in having sleep apnea. Today, the Reggie White Sleep Disorders Research and Education Foundation in Wisconsin works to educate the public to raise awareness about sleep apnea.

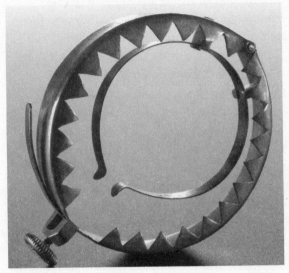

Jugum Penis, steel, nickel plated, employed on young men during sleep in the 1800s to prevent impure thoughts.

Impure Thoughts

David's story: Before the days of Viagra, we would do sleep studies to differentiate between organic and psychological impotence (today called ED). If the problem was organic, the treatment might involve surgery, but the surgical option wouldn't be recommended unless there were no other alternatives. A sleep study could help make the proper diagnosis. Since men get erections during stage REM sleep, and since these erections are independent of dream content and are a physiological response, if a man can achieve an erection during sleep but not during wakefulness, it implies that the cause of his problem is psychological. In that case, he would not need surgery and could, instead, opt for a psychological treatment.

I always thought that if you didn't have a psychological problem with impotence prior to the sleep study, you probably would after the test. We prepared the patient by putting a strain gauge on his penis prior to the study. During REM sleep, a technician would watch the strain gauges for any indication of an erection. When the gauge appeared to be at a maximum, the technician would go in to the room, pull back the covers, and take a photograph! They would then calculate the bending strength of the penis. That seemed a little traumatic to me. The home version of this test was to glue postage stamps tightly around the flaccid penis prior to bedtime. In the morning, if the stamps broke, it was assumed you had an erection. Viagra and other medical treatments diminished the value of these tests.

During Victorian times, it was thought that the erections young boys had during sleep were related to impure thoughts. A device called the Jugum Penis was invented around 1880 to help these boys avoid such thoughts. It was a metal clip that fit snugly on the penis. Around the clips were a set of barbs like saw teeth. If the penis enlarged, it would contact the barbs and awaken the sleeper, thus sparing him the danger of impure thoughts.

RESTLESS LEGS SYNDROME

Restless legs syndrome (RLS) is described as an irresistible need to move or stretch the legs. The sensation occurs primarily at bedtime but may also occur when sedentary during the day. About 20 percent of patients describe it as painful, but it's not cramping, like with a charley horse. Movement will temporarily relieve the discomfort. This disorder can make it very difficult to fall asleep at night and may prolong awakenings during the night. The level of discomfort can vary night to night, with some nights being symptom-free. There may be a relationship between RLS and low iron. Ferritin levels should be checked if there is suspicion of the disorder.[11]

RLS is known to run in some families. Several genes are associated with the condition.[12] Women often first notice RLS during pregnancy, and it usually goes away following the birth of the child. The disorder is more common in women but can occur in men and can also occur at almost any age. Growing pains in children may be an indication of RLS.

About 70 percent of people with RLS also have another condition called periodic limb movements during sleep (PLMS). These are described as twitches or kicks of the legs and sometimes the arms that occur repetitively during sleep. Sufferers often come to the clinic with a complaint of sleep maintenance insomnia: "I can get to sleep; I just keep waking up." The afflicted individual is usually unaware of the twitching. About 25 percent of cases are referred by a bed partner whose sleep was disturbed by the movement. If you have RLS, there's a high probability you also have PLMS. However, you can have PLMS without the RLS component. Like RLS, PLMS can be quite variable. It can change from nonexistent one night to severe the next. Sleep studies can be used to detect the presence of the limb movements. However, some people have frequent limb movements that don't seem to interfere with sleep. When patients come to us, the sleep lab will count the number of limb movements and calculate a PLM index (number of limb movements per hour of sleep). The sleep center will also count how many of the limb movements led to arousal and will calculate a PLM arousal index. If limb movements aren't causing arousals, treatment is generally not recommended. Treatment for PLMS is very similar to RLS. The same medications are used.

Tips for treating RLS. It is a good idea to seek medical treatment if your RLS is causing you to lose sleep. The type of doctor you see first could be your family doctor, or you could go directly to a sleep lab and request a consultation for the condition. Since it is a problem that we see all the time in the clinic, the sleep expert will be able to help you diagnose the severity of the condition and help you deal with it.

Sometimes the condition can be alleviated by eliminating alcohol, caffeine, nicotine, or other foods or drugs. Other times the condition will resolve after underlying diseases are treated, such as diabetes, thyroid disorders, or kidney disease. Although a number of pharmaceutical drugs are also available to treat the condition, some physicians, such as Carolyn Dean and Andrew Weil, have found that magnesium works to alleviate the problem.

According to a National Sleep Foundation poll, 80 percent of US adults have not talked with their doctor about their sleep.

NARCOLEPSY

Narcolepsy has been written about in scientific literature for over a hundred years. It was first described by Jean-Baptiste-Édouard Gélineau (1828–1906), a French physician. The word "narcolepsy" comes from a combination of two Greek words, *narke*, meaning "stupor" or "numbness," and *lepsis*, meaning "attack" or "seizure." Narcolepsy is a neurological disorder in which the sufferer experiences increased drowsiness and is prone to fall asleep suddenly. These incidents are called sleep attacks. However, with more refined assessment abilities, many people previously diagnosed with narcolepsy find they actually have another sleep disorder, such as sleep apnea. A number of symptoms correspond with narcolepsy. These include:

Sleep paralysis. Mentally waking up but being completely unable to move. Usually described as frightening and generally lasting only a few seconds to minutes.

Hypnagogic hallucinations. Vivid auditory or visual hallucinations that typically occur during the onset of sleep. Most people report them during the night or during sedentary times of the day.

Daytime sleepiness. This is the primary symptom that leads to treatment. While the quality of the sleepiness can vary,[13] many narcoleptics talk about sleep attacks. These are described as episodes where the person feels relatively alert, followed quickly by an intense need to sleep. They may nap for only a few minutes, but this brief nap can prove very refreshing. These sleep attacks may happen several times a day. This is differentiated from the sleepiness of an apnea patient who describes sleepiness as more pervasive during the day and for whom short naps are not refreshing.

Disrupted nocturnal sleep. Narcoleptics have the worst of both worlds. They are very sleepy during the day, yet they sleep very poorly at night.

Cataplexy. A rapid loss of muscle tone associated with an emotion. The most common trigger for cataplexy is laughter. With the emotion, the muscles can stop working and the individual can fall to the ground or slump in a chair. They do not lose consciousness. This symptom occurs only with narcolepsy. No other sleep disorder causes it. All the other symptoms can also be caused by other sleep disorders.

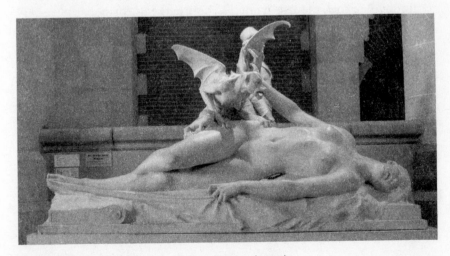

The Nightmare. *Sculpture by Eugène Thivier (1894).*

Only about 10 to 15 percent of people with narcolepsy demonstrate all of these symptoms. The majority have only some of the symptoms. The prevalence of narcolepsy is about 0.05 percent of the US population. It affects about 0.18 percent of the population of Japan and is very rare in Israel (0.02 percent). It tends to affect men more than women. The peak age of onset of narcolepsy is during the teenage years to early twenties. It often takes years between the onset of symptoms and making a diagnosis.

A recent study found that individuals with narcolepsy have lost neurons in a portion of the hypothalamus that produces a chemical called hypocretin or orexin (it has two names because it was discovered simultaneously at two universities: Stanford and the University of Texas Southwestern Medical School). Treatment of narcolepsy typically involves the use of medications, often multiple to control all of the symptoms. For example, the sleepiness component requires the use of stimulant medications; the disturbed sleep component may require a hypnotic medication; and the cataplexy, sleep paralysis, and hypnagogic hallucinations may require an antidepressant. A relatively new medication, sodium oxybate, improves sleep at night, greatly reduces cataplexy, and enhances daytime alertness. The recent discovery of the loss of hypocretin neurons may lead to the development of new medications to target that specific area of the brain.

Jimmy Kimmel, the late-night TV host and comedian, has been very open about his struggle with narcolepsy. The forty-three-year-old wasn't diagnosed with the disorder until he was in his thirties. Talking about his ailment in an interview with *Esquire,* he said he finally went to a doctor after he began to require gallons of iced tea to get through the afternoon. When describing the condition, Kimmel likened the disorder to someone gently sitting on his brain—just the inside of his head being tired. According to some sources, out of the estimated two hundred thousand Americans who suffer from narcolepsy, fewer than fifty thousand are diagnosed.

Sleep Bulimia: Binging on sleep over the weekend

To be your very best in bed, be alert for signs and symptoms of sleep disorders. Unrecognized and untreated sleep disorders will impede success and erode performance on all levels, both individually and organizationally. If left untreated, these disorders can stress the body and lead to a variety of physical and psychological problems, some of which are quite serious. Most people are poor judges at gauging how well they sleep, and that is where sleep lab data can be extremely useful. The majority of sleep disorders can be successfully treated, resulting in improved health, optimum functioning, peak performance, and an enhanced quality of life.

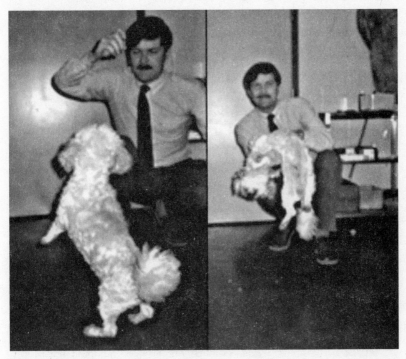

This is my colleague Dr. Andrew Jamieson performing an experiment with a dog that has cataplexy, a sudden loss of muscle tone associated with an emotion. When it got excited after receiving a treat, it became paralyzed.

When to See a Sleep Specialist

Your primary care physician may refer you to a sleep specialist, or your bed partner may insist on it when they can't sleep because of your snoring. In most cases, you don't need a referral to see a sleep specialist.

You may find that your sleep is not leaving you restored or refreshed upon awakening. It is not normal to wake up feeling exhausted. Common and valid reasons to seek help from a sleep specialist include the inability to fall asleep or stay asleep, waking too early, and excessive daytime sleepiness. Do you fall asleep while sitting still, reading, or watching television? Other reasons may include awakening during the night gasping or choking, waking with your heart pounding, having trouble concentrating during the day, morning headaches, depression, irritability, sexual dysfunction, and memory difficulties.

A sleep specialist is either in the medical or psychology field. Individuals who completed the required training and experience and successfully passed the certification examinations administered by the American Board of Sleep Medicine (ABSM) are referred to as diplomates of the American Board of Sleep Medicine. Practitioners who pass the ABSM board have the DABSM (Diplomate of the American Board of Sleep Medicine) credential. Those who pass the Behavioral Sleep Medicine certification exam have the credential CBSM (Certified in Behavioral Sleep Medicine). The ABSM website, www.absm.org, lists certified practitioners. The American Academy of Sleep Medicine and the National Sleep Foundation websites list sleep specialists and accredited sleep centers. Sleep technologists have the credential RPSGT (Registered Polysomnographic Technologist) and are also listed at www.absm.org. Nurse practitioners, registered nurses, and physician assistants also practice within the specialty. Specialized help is available for sleep questions, problems, and to improve your sleep. Valuing and protecting your sleep health and wellness will serve to maximize your potential, increase your achievements, and extend your successes.

CHAPTER FIFTEEN

SLEEP, DRUGS, AND ROCK & ROLL

If it wasn't for the coffee, I'd have no identifiable personality whatsoever.

—David Letterman

Psychoactive substances abound in nature, and even before we started popping pills, we were chewing coca leaves and gnawing iboga root bark to get into an altered state. It's definitely a human thing. Hypnos, the jovial little Greek god of sleep, is often pictured with an armful of poppies. He obviously had connections. The ability to ferment grains, juice, and honey has been around for thousands of years. Sleeping pills may be relative newcomers to the psychoactive party, but they're already a multibillion dollar industry. They're also a clear indication of the widespread prevalence of sleep problems. And, yes, there are substances to help us sleep and to keep us awake.

ALCOHOL

It's really astonishing how many people resort to self-medicating with alcohol to help them fall asleep. However, the chronic use of alcohol doesn't improve sleep. Instead, it can very quickly become the source of sleep problems.

Infrequent and modest alcohol consumption within three hours of bedtime may in fact help a person fall asleep more quickly, and it is one of the few substances that can increase stage 3 NREM sleep. This fact may be why people feel that alcohol improves sleep: they fall asleep more quickly and it is deeper. However, the positive effects of alcohol on sleep last only a few hours. During the latter portion of the night, there are more awakenings as alcohol is metabolized. Alcohol may also suppress REM sleep early in the night, and that sleep stage can "rebound" during the latter portion of the sleep cycle. When REM is suppressed, it's as if the body knows it's not getting enough of this essential sleep stage. When it's no longer suppressed, it will come back with a vengeance. REM sleep will rebound by occurring more than the normal amount, which is the brain's way of trying to make up for the lost sleep stage. This type of REM rebound can result in unpleasant dreams and nightmares.

> Alcohol isn't a particularly good short- or long-term solution to sleep problems.

Alcohol also selectively decreases muscle tone in the tongue and throat, which narrows the upper airway. This is why some people snore after drinking. And some snorers develop sleep apnea after consuming alcohol. People with preexisting obstructive sleep apnea can experience worsening of their condition with alcohol use. After just a few nights of drinking, the alcohol's positive benefits of hastening sleep onset and increasing stage 3 NREM sleep are lost. However, the negative effects persist. The sleep of alcoholics is quite disrupted, and increasingly higher doses of alcohol may be required to get any sleep benefit at all.

Alcohol isn't a particularly good short- or long-term solution to sleep problems. Still, the negative effects of alcohol on sleep don't mean that one must quit drinking entirely. A glass of wine at dinner has no significant effect on sleep, yet several glasses of wine within three hours of bedtime can certainly contribute to sleep problems. There is really no role for alcohol in treating sleep problems or even helping a person fall asleep. Even with acute use, the negatives far outweigh the positives.

It's important to note that sleep deprivation and alcohol use will interact. After five nights of partial sleep deprivation, three alcoholic drinks will have the same effect on your cognitive ability and reaction time as six drinks would when you've slept enough. If a person can normally function well with one to two glasses of wine, they may be functionally intoxicated with those same two drinks if they're even modestly sleep deprived. There is a tendency in this country to curtail sleep during the workweek and then to go out Friday night to happy hour. Sleep-deprived individuals consuming alcohol will double the impairment level of each drink, which is potentially a scenario for disaster.

OUR COFFEE CULTURE

"Sleep is a symptom of caffeine deprivation," said some anonymous wit. Without question, caffeine is the most commonly used stimulant in the world, and coffee is the second most traded commodity in the world. Caffeine is also found in sodas (both cola and non-cola), chocolate, energy drinks (even some energy water), weight-loss pills, pain relievers, some breath fresheners, and over-the-counter as well as prescription medications. The highest concentration of caffeine in the blood is achieved within fifteen minutes to two hours after consumption. It takes between two and a half to four and a half hours for half of the drug to be eliminated.[1] This means that the effects of caffeine can last for several hours.

The primary effects that caffeine has on sleep are to lengthen the time it takes to fall asleep and to decrease the total amount of sleep obtained. Most people experience these effects for three to four hours following consumption, but in caffeine-sensitive individuals, the negative effects can persist for much longer. Some people appear to develop a tolerance to the stimulating effects and can fall asleep quickly following consumption, with little apparent effect on their sleep. However, even in these individuals, caffeine may increase the lighter sleep stages and increase awakenings during the night. Generally caffeine doses of 100 to 150 mg (one cup of coffee) are required to produce the stimulant effects on sleep. However, doses as small as 32 mg have been shown to influence sleep and alertness. This is the level of caffeine present in most caffeinated sodas.

I have patients who consume several cups of coffee in the evenings prior to bedtime. When I make this observation, they say, "Dr. Brown, coffee does not bother my sleep." I counter with, "But you are not sleeping." The response: "Yes, but it's not the coffee."

> Caffeine doesn't provide any of the restorative properties of sleep that will help you think clearly.

Most people with sleep problems are well aware of the negative effects of caffeine on sleep. Yet we're always amazed at how often people are consuming high levels of caffeine and still complaining about their sleep. One of our patients told us that she typically kept a liter of Mountain Dew on her bedside table every night, and during the course of the evening she would consume the entire bottle. This amounts to 304 mg of caffeine. When asked about the soda, she claimed that the caffeine wasn't the source of her problem. She was wrong: the real issue was that she liked Mountain Dew and had no intention of giving it up for the sake of her sleep. Another patient downed her sleeping pills at night with a cup of coffee.

Caffeine works by blocking adenosine receptors, a chemical in the brain that makes us feel sleepy. As a result, we feel less sleepy. However, caffeine doesn't provide any of the restorative properties of sleep that will help you think clearly, function optimally, or maintain good health.[2] If you're having sleep problems, be careful about caffeine and back down on its use. Keep it as far away from bedtime as possible, and make certain you're not inadvertently consuming it in over-the-counter or prescription medication.

Caffeine abuse and dependence may be becoming more common as we continue to put off the sleep we so desperately need. The latest edition of the Diagnostic and Statistical Manual of Mental Disorders (the DSM) has provisions for caffeine-related disorders, including caffeine intoxication and caffeine withdrawal. For instance, if you consume more than 250 mg of caffeine and experience five or more of the following symptoms, you may have caffeine intoxication: restlessness, nervousness, excitement, insomnia, flushed face, diuresis, gastrointestinal upset, muscle twitching, rambling flow of thought or speech, rapid or irregular heartbeat, periods of inexhaustibility or psychomotor agitation. Fatigue, difficulty focusing, and headache are listed as symptoms of caffeine withdrawal.

The American Association of Poison Control Centers is now tracking energy drink overdoses and side effects.

ENERGY DRINKS

So-called energy drinks are the fastest-growing segment of the beverage market, especially among teens and young adults. Can this market share be attributed to our lack of sleep? Similar to coffee, and often containing caffeine, energy drinks are commonly perceived as stimulating performance enhancers. However, caffeine toxicity and adverse events have been reported with excessive consumption, and different formulations and ingredients have unknown safety profiles that can be dangerous, if not lethal. The most common adverse events affect the neurological and cardiovascular systems. Energy drink consumption is also linked to risk-taking behaviors and substance abuse. The combination of energy drinks and alcohol is especially worrisome and may be riskier than alcohol alone, placing the user at a higher risk for binge drinking, high-risk driving behaviors, and dependence.

Stay Awake, Alert, and Productive Naturally

Nothing replaces sufficient sleep, but here are some alerting strategies that come in handy for afternoon energy slumps.

- Move around, exercise, or take a walk.
- Get fresh air and sunlight.
- Turn on bright lights.
- Practice deep breathing.
- Stay hydrated.
- Stand up.
- Have a healthy snack.
- Chew gum or ice.
- Watch a funny video.
- Listen to upbeat music.
- Try aromatherapy: peppermint oil, rosemary, eucalyptus, and cinnamon are all alerting scents.
- Drink rosemary tea.
- Take a nap. If that isn't possible, close your eyes for five to ten minutes and rest.

Bear in mind that nothing will replace sufficient sleep, and drowsy driving should be avoided at all costs since involuntary and uncontrollable microsleeps will occur in the face of sleep loss.

CIGARETTES

Nicotine is another psychoactive drug and a major

arette smoke. Cigarettes typically contain between ⌐.⌐

nicotine. Nicotine can negatively affect sleep during use and upon with-drawal. Due to nicotine's short half-life, a smoker wakes each morning in withdrawal. As we have seen with some clinic patients, this withdrawal can occur in the middle of the night. It comes as no surprise (and is con-firmed by the research) that sleep quality is worse in people who smoke cigarettes. Cigarette smoking has been associated with insomnia-like symptoms, such as trouble falling asleep, difficulty staying asleep, strug-gling to wake up, and even nightmares and daytime sleepiness. In addi-tion, B.A. Philips and F.J. Danner found that smokers reported minor accidents, depression, and high daily caffeine intake more so than non-smokers. Another study by D. Revicki found that smokers were more likely than nonsmokers to sleep less than six hours a night. Smoking is also associated with sleep-related respiratory disorders.

> Marilyn Monroe died from an overdose of sleeping pills at the age
> of thirty-six.

OVER-THE-COUNTER SLEEPING PILLS

The FDA began to review over-the-counter (OTC) drugs in the 1970s. Though most people consider OTC sleeping medications safe, these drugs do have side effects and can be long acting, causing morning sedation and impairing driving. They can also produce anticholiner-gic effects (dry eyes and mouth, and difficulty urinating) and cognitive pairment persisting into the day following nighttime use. They're not recommended for the elderly since the anticholinergic effects can cause confusion and forgetfulness. Tolerance to these medications develops quickly and they typically lose their effectiveness with long-term use. The biggest advantage of OTC sleeping pills is that you don't need a prescription. However, they can be more dangerous than some prescription medications. It might be a good idea to talk with your doctor about these medications even though no prescription is needed.

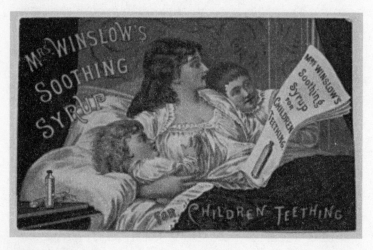

Mrs. Winslow's Soothing Syrup, a morphine–alcohol patent medicine for babies. In the 1840s, druggists Jeremiah Curtis and Benjamin A. Perkins manufactured an interesting concoction advertised for helping teething babies and "producing natural, quiet sleep" that was created by Curtis's mother-in-law. The two primary ingredients were morphine and alcohol. Curtis reported selling more than 1.5 million bottles of the remedy annually, which was sold as late as 1930. The American Medical Times *described the syrup as a baby killer, noting that parents were "relieved of all further care of their infants" through its use.*

Melatonin is important for shutting down the circadian alerting rhythms that would otherwise keep you awake.

MELATONIN

Melatonin is a hormone produced by the body's pineal gland, located just above the middle of the brain. During the day the production of melatonin is inhibited, but when the sun sets and darkness occurs, the pineal gland begins to actively produce this hormone, which is released into the bloodstream. As a result, melatonin levels in the blood rise sharply, and you begin to feel less alert and eventually become sleepy. Melatonin is primarily a body clock regulator, not a sleep initiator. It works with your biological clock by telling your brain when it is time to sleep. But the hormone does not increase your sleep drive or need for sleep. Instead, melatonin is important for shutting down the circadian alerting rhythms that would otherwise keep you awake despite the presence of a strong sleep drive (see "The Two Factors of Sleep Control" on page 19).

In pill form, melatonin doesn't function like your body's naturally produced hormone. Taken as a supplement, it affects the brain in bursts and rapidly leaves the system as a result of its short half-life, unlike the slow buildup and washout of naturally produced melatonin. Children produce a great deal of melatonin but the amount drops with puberty. Interestingly, the pineal gland also shrinks during this time. As we get older, some people continue to produce high levels of melatonin while others produce less. This may explain why some people respond to supplemental melatonin with improved sleep while others don't.

Melatonin is useful in treating jet lag. It's best to take it after dark the day you travel, and also after dark for a few days after arriving at your destination. The supplement can also cause mild side effects in some people: 2 to 3 mg can produce sleepiness, headaches, next-day grogginess, nausea, changes in blood pressure, vivid dreams, nightmares, and hormone fluctuations.

Until the invention of the electric light, it was thought that humans didn't experience nighttime lights bright enough to significantly suppress melatonin secretion. Today, in contrast, we live in an unnatural, light-polluted environment that's arguably causing significant harm. We suppress melatonin secretion with modern lights, depriving ourselves of the hormone's numerous benefits. Melatonin is a strong anticancer agent and it boosts the immune system. Shift work is an independent risk factor for many cancers, possibly because of the loss of melatonin. It turns out that the light most likely to suppress melatonin is in the blue wavelengths. If you're having trouble sleeping, be very aware of light, particularly in the evening hours.

Alcohol and sleeping pills proved a lethal combination, causing the death of Brian Epstein, the Beatles' manager, in 1967 at the age of thirty-two.

THE BOTTOM LINE

Caffeine, energy drinks, cigarette smoking, and stimulants can contribute to poor sleep quality. For this reason you should exercise care when using these products. If you want to get the maximum return for the time you invest in sleeping, it is prudent to limit stimulants. There are an array of medications and substances that can benefit and hinder sleep, but to date, nothing has been found that can duplicate the restorative biological benefits of sleep or compensate for a lack of sleep.

We are not certain. But it looks like sleeping pills could be as risky as smoking cigarettes. It looks much more dangerous to take these pills than to treat insomnia another way.

—DR. DANIEL F. KRIPKE, emeritus professor of psychiatry
at the University of California

ARE SLEEPING PILLS DANGEROUS?

Sleeping pills evoke quite mixed reactions both in medical and patient communities. Some physicians and patients will do anything to avoid them, while others don't question the need to take them nightly. While it appears that newer sleeping agents have less addiction potential than their predecessors, dependency remains an issue that must be considered with these drugs.

Any medication that causes sedation can create problems when you are driving or engaging in other potentially dangerous activities if they're in your system at the time of the activity. This includes over-the-counter medications, which can be longer acting than many prescription medications.

Some sleep researchers, including Dr. Daniel Kripke at the University of California, have raised other concerns with sleeping pills. In a study of more than thirty-four thousand people, he found that those who took prescription sleeping medication, even occasionally, had a 5.3-fold higher death risk and a 35 percent higher risk of cancer compared to nonusers. Critics point out that his study simply showed a correlation with sleeping pill use, not a causal relationship. They note that sicker people also have more sleep problems and so are more likely to use sleeping pills.

This area of investigation remains controversial, and hopefully additional studies will clarify the issue.[3]

CHAPTER SIXTEEN

SLEEPING WITH THE ENEMY

The stress of a day of hard work can make you sleep like a log
or it can keep you awake all night.

—Hans Selye, *The Stress of Life* (1956)

Probably the most meticulous investigator of biological stress was Hans Selye (1907–1982), a Hungarian scientist who conducted his laboratory work in Canada. His book *The Stress of Life* (1956) is a classic investigation of the causes of stress and the mechanisms by which it operates to impair, and sometimes repair, the body. Selye begins the volume with one of the clearest summaries of what stress is, and his definition will be useful as we look at the relationship between stress and sleep.

> In its medical sense, stress is essentially the rate of wear and tear in the body. Anyone who feels that whatever he is doing—or whatever is being done to him—is strenuous and wearing, knows vaguely what we mean by stress. The feelings of just being tired, jittery, or ill are subjective sensations of stress.[1]

He went on to observe that "stress is not necessarily something bad."[2] For example, you can experience stress from lifting weights in the gym, but such stress is good since it leads to stronger muscles. Selye discovered that in response to stress, the pituitary gland produces adrenocorticotrophic hormone (ACTH), which, in turn, incites the cells of the adrenal cortex—part of the adrenal gland, a hormone-producing endocrine gland attached to the top of each kidney—to produce corticoids. Corticoids are steroid hormones.

The important message that Selye underscored for us relates to the effect of stress on the biological organism. It is a physical effect, and it can cause damage throughout the body.

SLEEP AND STRESS

Since the purpose of this book is to help you succeed by getting quality sleep, it's important to look at the relationship between stress and sleep. The reason for this focus on stress should be obvious. As Dr. Selye explained, stress can often result in a generalized whole-body response, and that wear and tear can have a profound negative impact on our ability to function. It's important for anyone who wants to succeed to know how to deal with stress.

Stress and sleep affect one another: that is, the relationship is bidirectional. If you get insufficient sleep, you'll experience stress. And if you're stressed by anything negative, such as the loss of a job or conflict with a loved one, you can expect to experience sleep disturbances.

It follows from this analysis—and the research studies back up this conclusion—that by reducing stress in your life, you will improve your sleep. At the same time, by getting better sleep, you will reduce stress.

Selye had a good sense of humor, and when asked how he dealt with stress in his own life, he said, "I thrive on stress. I like to work a lot."

That's positive stress. But what about negative stress, the kind that could keep you up at night? We're going to discuss how to reduce that kind of stress in your life. Even though some stress can be beneficial for you (such as exercising, falling in love, or working), we'll focus on how to eliminate negative stress, the kind that can build up an overabundance of hormones like cortisol and adrenaline, leading to a stress response.

HOW TO REDUCE STRESS

There are many effective ways to reduce stress. In our practice, we've found the following activities can work for various patients. Each of these methods has been employed successfully by many people to reduce stress and lead to better sleep.

- Meditation
- Yoga
- Exercise
- Putting work out of mind
- Creative artwork, such as coloring, painting, writing, and drawing
- Music, either playing it or listening to it
- Walking
- Journaling
- Sex
- Napping
- Light reading
- Guided imagery

Although we've found that these techniques are quite effective, it's true that all people are different, so not everything will work with everyone. In fact, some people are simply more predisposed to sleep problems. This is due to environment, upbringing, and genetics, just as some people are more predisposed to certain physical ills, such as heart problems, cancer, or high blood pressure. People also differ in their ability to tolerate stress: some have a low tolerance for almost any stress while others have a high tolerance. Remember, Hans Selye said he enjoyed the stress of working, and over the course of his career he published 1,700 scientific articles. Regardless, given enough stress, all of us will develop sleep problems.

> The ability to adopt and sustain a regular normal sleep schedule may be the single most important aspect enabling us to level the playing field and increase the quality of our lives.
> —MICHELLE SMITH, "Stress and Sleep Deprivation" (2013)

One of the chief sources of stress for people with insomnia is that their minds are overly active, especially at night. This thinking can keep them up into the wee hours. There are two approaches to dealing with overthinking. The first solution is to use guided imagery (see page 150) to calm the mind. The second approach is to realize that nighttime problems are always exaggerated. When we get in bed at night and we're stuck with our thoughts, it can be difficult to let the world and its problems go so that sleep can overtake us. This is essentially a control issue. In other words, overthinking and anxiety are methods of trying to control our world. If I think about it long enough, I can anticipate every possible negative outcome and will not be surprised when more bad things happen to me. Historically, this kind of hypervigilance had survival value for early humans. It caused our ancestors to believe there was a lion behind a bush at the slightest rustling of the leaves, for example. We have inherited this trait. But what is the actual likelihood that a lion is really present? Yes, it would be disastrous if it were but unless you live in a zoo, today it's very unlikely that this will be the case. To use a more contemporary example, you hear a noise at night and your immediate response is that someone has broken into the house intent on causing you harm. While that's a possible cause of the noise, it could also be your child getting a glass of water, the dog turning over, or the house settling in the coolness of the night. It's okay to think the worst—that's the gift of our ancestors—but in many situations you can use the power of logic to back off from the worst-case scenario and come to a more realistic assessment of the situation.

SLEEP TRUMPS STRESS

Remember that one of Hans Selye's biggest discoveries about stress was that negative stress can produce a systemic increase in certain hormones, specifically ACTH, cortisol, and adrenaline. This can lead to a crisis where the body has too much of these hormones. Therefore, if there was some way to reduce this general system-wide stress response, it could help the body cope with stress.

Well, wouldn't you know it—it just so happens that when we fall asleep, certain interesting chemical reactions occur in our brains and bodies. These reactions are exactly what we need to reduce excess levels of stress hormones. In fact, the same chemical that brings on slow wave sleep— the deepest level of slumber—also functions to reduce ACTH. In other words, as the body slides deeper into slumberland, a kind of biological switch is activated inside us to reduce stress. And the value of sleep is not just the fact that we're relaxed and unconscious. There's actually a switch that appears to shut down ACTH overload for us, so that stress is lessened in a measurable way. We experience reduced levels of ACTH, which in turn reduces cortisol and adrenaline, inducing relaxation and calmness.

The biological switch inside our brain is called a corticotropin inhibiting factor (CIF). This chemical shuts down the excess ACTH being churned out by our overworked and overstressed adrenals. Although the exact agent hasn't been definitively isolated yet in humans, we know it must be there because of the chemical reactions that occur when we sleep: this agent (most likely a peptide) causes us to descend into slow wave sleep.[3] While we're in that wonderful realm, we physically experience a deep calm as stress is eliminated.

The example that follows may sound a bit silly, but it was a real scientific study to reduce stress in mice and it illustrates an important concept. Now, you may know that mice are used in biological tests all the time because they're rather similar to humans genetically. So if something works in a mouse, it's likely to work in humans; at least, it's more likely to work in people than something tested in a rabbit, for instance, or a trout.

So, to stress out the mice, the scientists stepped on their feet. Once the mice were basically saying things like "Ouch!" and "Bejabbers!" and "What the heck did you do that for!" and after the mice had experienced high levels of stress as a result of getting their tiny little feet stepped on by big human researchers, then, and only then, did the scientists do right by those little mice by injecting a peptide into their bodies that calmed them down, soothed their nerves, and basically reduced the stress and insult they had received from their keepers. This peptide eliminated the ACTH stress response.[4]

What does this experiment mean for you? It means a whole lot since we now know that we can stop stress in its tracks with a peptide, and that the same peptide is released when we sleep. This fundamental point is worth repeating. We can stop stress in its tracks with deep sleep. Yes, good sleep will wipe out the stressors of the previous day. It will wipe the slate clean, so to speak, and ensure that you wake up feeling refreshed and ready to tackle the world anew. Bright eyed and bushy tailed.

So, next time you get your feet stepped on by someone, don't let the stress build up to intolerable levels. Don't stay up all night thinking about it. Instead, do what those mice did. Get a good night's sleep, and experience the soothing relief from your own brain chemicals and adrenal glands. Let your body flip the switch inside your head. Experience the deep, satisfying relief that can only come from deep sleep.

You deserve to feel as calm as a Buddhist monk. Why not come right out and admit that you deserve to sleep like a baby? That's the goal of all who desire good sleep. After all, if you could get that kind of restful sleep—and you can!—what a wonderful thing it would be. You'd wake up refreshed and unstressed. All the angst would be gone. You would be ready to face the world like a champion.

This, then, is what sleep—good sleep, the kind of sleep we're talking about in this book—is all about. Rest. Relaxation. Wiping the slate clean.

And now we know that these aren't just words and ideas. Thanks to Hans Selye and the researchers who followed in his footsteps, we know that a chemical cascade really does take place when we're asleep. A beautiful symphony of biological compounds. It will put out the fires burning in your brain. It will ease your troubled mind. It will make things good again, just as if no one had ever stepped on your foot after all.

CHAPTER SEVENTEEN

HOW ABOUT A QUICKIE?

With great power comes a great need to take a nap. Wake me up later.

—Rick Riordan, *The Last Olympian* (2009)

If you happen to live in Ador, Spain, you probably consider yourself lucky. The mayor of that town, which is near the east coast of the country, recently made a very important announcement. In July 2015, Mayor Joan Faus Vitoria issued a proclamation that created an official nap time for the entire city.

"From now on," the mayor effectively said, "everyone in this city will observe a common nap time from 2:00 p.m. to 5:00 p.m. each day. During this time the town's inhabitants, as well as visitors and tourists, are encouraged to take their afternoon siesta. The reason for this law is that it's very hot during the afternoon, and it's best if people don't work."

Mayor Vitoria is a jovial-looking chap who resembles Bob Keeshan, the creator of Captain Kangaroo. "No, don't worry, I'm not making it a law that requires people to sleep," he explained. "It's more of a suggestion. But we want people to keep the noise level down during this time period, so that workers in their shops and people in their homes who wish to take a nap can do so without disturbance."

If you need any more evidence of the validity of napping, look no further than this forward-thinking town official. With one fell swoop of his pen, he became the first mayor in Spain to codify the national custom of taking a nap during the afternoon. His new legislation is informed by the huge amount of data on the value of naps.

ARE NAPS A GOOD WAY TO MAKE UP FOR LOST SLEEP?

The short answer is yes, but they may not be the *best* way to do this. As we have previously observed, probably the best way to make up for lost sleep is to get two or more nights of quality sleep.[1] But failing that, naps have a high intrinsic value for most people.[2]

One of the negative things that happens when you're sleep deprived, even for a few hours, is that your body produces excess norepinephrine, a biological compound that puts stress on the heart and raises blood pressure. Naps effectively prevent this excess production of norepinephrine, reducing stress on your heart and vascular system.[3] Sleep deprivation also causes unfavorable changes in Interleukin-6, a protein that can cause inflammation and disrupt the immune system. Naps prevent this unfavorable condition, and in doing so bolster your immune system.[4] They also foster a healthy cardiovascular system and reduce your risk of debilitating heart failure.[5]

Many studies call specific attention to sanctioned naps as a way to boost work performance. Air traffic controllers, who must be eternally vigilant, were studied with and without a forty-minute nap. Even though the sanctioned nap at work was short and shallow, it still resulted in a significant improvement in objective measures of alertness and performance for this critical job.[6]

> There is more refreshment and stimulation in a nap, even of the briefest, than in all the alcohol ever distilled.
>
> —OVID

SLEEP INERTIA

When we awaken, whether from a night of sleep or a nap, we experience a period of grogginess and disorientation. During this interlude of foggy thinking and impaired motor control—which may last from a few minutes to half an hour or more—we are not exactly fit to operate heavy machinery, drive a car, or make critical business decisions. This period of impaired mental and physical functioning is called sleep inertia.

Naturally, if you take a sanctioned nap on the job, you'll have to be mindful of the effects of sleep inertia. Some researchers have suggested that sleep inertia is only a problem if the nap is more than half an hour long.[7] This may be due to the sleep stage that you enter. In a short fifteen- to twenty-minute nap, the likelihood is that you'll stay in stage 2 sleep. If you sleep longer, you may sink into stage 3 sleep, a very deep sleep stage. When you awaken out of stage 3 sleep, you'll be groggy and disoriented, and this feeling can last thirty to forty-five minutes. While a longer nap may have more recuperative value, a brief nap can recharge your batteries for at least a short period of time and it can avoid sleep inertia.

Sleep inertia from a nap can be worsened when combined with prior sleep deprivation. If you've been chronically sleep deprived, you'll probably drop into stage 3 sleep quickly, even during a short nap. The more sleep deprived you are, the worse the sleep inertia will be—regardless of the length of your nap. Others have noted that despite the disadvantages of sleep inertia—slower mental functioning and slightly impaired motor control—sanctioned naps still are preferable to operating with a sleep debt, especially for pilots.[8] Pilots? Yes, believe it or not, we'll have a lot more to say about the value (even for pilots) of sanctioned napping on the job.

> What happens during a ninety-minute nap that can turn a psychotic dwarf into a delightful two-year-old? That so dramatically alters the waking behavior of that child's brain that they go from being unbearable to totally delightful? I suspect that the same thing happens to adults, but we're so much trained and equipped to suppress our crankiness that it's less evident.
>
> —DR. ROBERT STICKGOLD

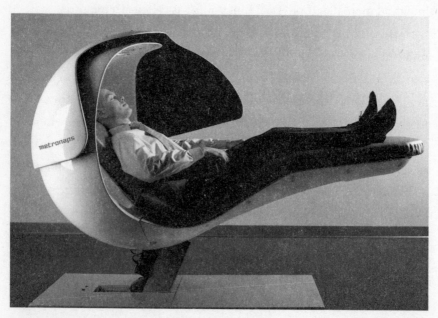

EnergyPod. Courtesy Nathan Sayers for MetroNaps.

COMBINING NAPS AND STIMULANTS

You might think that combining naps, which are inherently relaxing, with stimulants, which are energizing, might be a nonproductive idea, but people can get very sophisticated in how they hack their biology. For example, some savvy nappers will drink a cup of coffee and then immediately jump into bed to enjoy a quick nap. Since caffeine takes from fifteen to sixty minutes to kick in fully, they're able to sleep and refresh their cognitive and physical powers with a nap, and then when the caffeine hits them, they awaken with renewed mental clarity.

WHAT'S THE OPTIMUM LENGTH FOR A NAP?

Thomas Edison was notorious for taking naps at work. In fact, his sleeping style was so nap oriented he could be considered a nap fanatic. He used to boast to his employees that he didn't need a lot of sleep, and like Donald Trump he chided the mass of humanity for sleeping eight hours. But the great inventor operated under many mistaken notions, chief among them that you can get by on a reduced amount of sleep, and that people habitually overate and overslept because they were lazy.

Edison had a number of cots set up in his working environment, which allowed him to take naps whenever he was sleepy (fig. 4). We now know that taking short naps like this, even if you take them on the job, can work wonders for your mood, cognitive powers, and motor skills. Several researchers have demonstrated that napping for as little as ten minutes improves performance.[9] There's even evidence that shorter naps of seven to ten minutes confer recuperative effects, provided the sleeper manages to sink into stage 2 sleep.[10] Naps of less than thirty minutes'

duration confer several benefits, restoring wakefulness, promoting performance, boosting mood, and improving learning.[11]

It's speculated that short naps provide their benefits not by dissipat-
ing the sleep drive but rather by taking pressure off of the "sleep switch"
and allowing it to stay in the alert position longer.

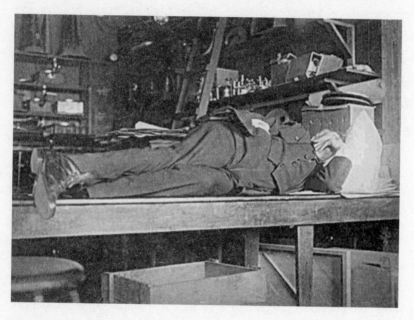

*Thomas Edison took many naps while working. Here he is pictured on a workbench,
taking a cat nap while wearing socks and shoes and a three-piece suit.*

POWER NAPS

A power nap is a short nap that ends before the sleeper enters deep sleep.
This avoids having the sleeper wake up in a groggy state. The term was
coined by Dr. James B. Maas, author of *Power Sleep* (1998) and emeritus
professor of Cornell's department of psychology. He was working with
IBM as a consultant at a time when power breakfasts and power lunches
were popular. So he said that rather than take a coffee or coke break, which
would interfere with nocturnal sleep, why not take a power nap?

Dr. Maas found that naps could have many beneficial effects on students and people in the workplace, restoring alertness and cognitive function. The key difference between an ordinary nap and a power nap is that with the latter you avoid the sleep inertia that can make you sluggish from a longer nap. It may sound counterintuitive to think that a shorter nap can promote more alertness, but this is exactly the case. And this is precisely why those who wish to increase their success during the workday should consider a power nap rather than a longer nap that would cause them to become sluggish.

The way to do a power nap is to set your alarm for thirty minutes. This ensures that you will not slip into the deepest stage of sleep. Instead, you will gain all the restorative energy from a short power nap while suffering none of the lethargy that comes with a nap that lasts for forty-five minutes or more. Power naps are especially helpful when traveling into new time zones, or before making an important presentation. As long as you keep these naps short, they will provide you with the energy you need to keep working for hours.

WHEN SHOULD YOU NAP?

Some evidence suggests that napping as soon as possible after you incur a sleep debt is best.[12] If you take a nap as soon as possible, you are more likely to revitalize your brain and body, improving your visual reaction time performance. It is also possible to nap prior to an expected sleep debt, putting sleep "into the bank" so that you prevent the serious impairment of brain and body that would otherwise occur with sleep deprivation.[13]

Our circadian rhythms may also help determine when it is a good time for a nap. As previously noted, the brain is activated during the day to counter the sleep drive. These alerting signals can become very strong in the evening, making sleep all but impossible (see sidebar on "The Two

Factors of Sleep Control," page 19). Interestingly, circadian alerting signals dip rather strongly in the midafternoon. The decreased alertness people typically feel after lunch may not be caused by a heavy meal or a boring meeting. It is physiological. Most people report feeling less alert from two to four in the afternoon. In fact, some cultural practices, such as the siesta, are designed around this time. Granted, the timing of siestas also corresponds to the hottest period of the day, but it's also the time when we're most likely to feel sleepy. You're also much more likely to make mistakes at this time of day. All types of accidents have increased rates of occurrence from midnight to 7:00 a.m. and between 2:00 and 4:00 in the afternoon, times that correspond with our highest levels of sleepiness. This midafternoon dip really is a good time to take a nap.

Taking a siesta may actually save your life. It has been known for some time that countries where siestas are popular have a lower incidence of coronary deaths. The late epidemiologist Dimitrios Trichopoulos studied more than twenty-three thousand Greek adults and looked at the relationship between napping and cardiac arrest. People who regularly and systematically napped were 37 percent less likely to die of coronary disease than nonnappers. Even occasional napping conferred a 12 percent decreased risk. The biggest benefit was received by working men who regularly took siestas: they enjoyed a 64 percent lower likelihood of dying from heart disease.

Keep in mind, too, that even short naps can be restorative. In other words, you don't have to drop all the way into slow wave sleep to benefit from a nap. So where are you expecting to get that little bit of extra sleep now? Not on the job, are you?

Or maybe that is a good idea after all . . .

Bill Gates admitted to napping under his desk during his early programming years.

SANCTIONED NAPPING ON THE JOB

Nurses do it . . . air traffic controllers do it . . . and now even pilots, for goodness sake—*pilots!*

Let me tell you something. Even though we know it's right, and that it works, it's still sometimes hard to believe that it's happening. I mean, a pilot sleeping while in the cockpit of a commercial airplane—hard to believe.

But despite the sleep inertia it causes, it has been found that allowing a pilot to take a short sanctioned snooze prior to landing, for example, will make the landing go better.[14] This whole concept—pilots enjoying a sanctioned nap—stems from the very real danger that can occur if a pilot is sleep deprived. When the captain takes a sanctioned nap, there's always another fully awake navigator or copilot at the controls, of course. But pilots have very difficult flight schedules, so they often find themselves short on sleep. Caffeine and other stimulants may help them stay awake, but as we have seen, stimulants are no substitute for restorative sleep. The bottom line is that "both researchers and pilots agree that the benefits associated with these naps far outweigh the potential risks."[15]

> "I'm going to examine the overhead panel."
> Pilot-speak for: "I'm going to take a nap."

Air traffic controllers also play a critical role in maintaining air safety. They must keep their attention focused on little dots of light moving across a screen, each of which represents an airplane full of people. In this high-stress position, failure is not an option. To discover how these pivotal people in the transportation industry functioned, researchers conducted a study in which fourteen air traffic controllers were allowed a forty-minute nap, and fourteen others worked straight through their shift. The researchers concluded that "although sleep taken at work is likely to be short and of poor quality, it still results in an improvement in objective measures of alertness and performance."[16] These words are a strong endorsement for the concept of allowing sanctioned naps on the job.

Along with pilots and air traffic controllers, night shift nurses also play a critical role in the lives of their patients. And like pilots and air traffic controllers, night shift nurses benefit from being allowed short naps while on duty. When tested, nurses who were allowed to nap at work did better on the psychomotor vigilance test (PVT).[17] Researchers concluded that "nighttime napping is an effective measure to prevent adverse effects due to night shift work."[18]

NAPS FOR SUCCESS

Bernie Williams was infamous for taking naps before going out to batting practice with the New York Yankees. These weren't sanctioned naps and he wasn't supposed to be sleeping in the clubhouse.[19] But that extra sleep helped him do his best. Well, now serious research backs up Bernie's approach to keeping his game sharp.

Ten healthy males were studied to determine the effect of an after-lunch nap on their athletic performance.[20] In some rather amazing findings, sprint time improved in a statistically significant amount for those who took the short naps. Naturally, these results have important implications for all athletes, including boxers, mountain climbers, and race car drivers. Some of these sports involve physical danger, and being able to perform at your best is critical not only for winning but also for staying alive. Anyone familiar with *Into Thin Air: A Personal Account of the Mt. Everest Disaster* (1997) knows as much.

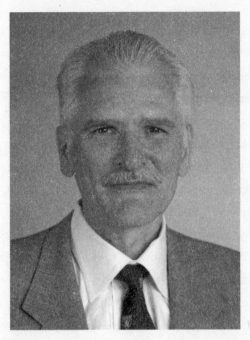

Dr. Charles Czeisler, affectionately known in the NBA as the "sleep doctor," advises athletes on how to use naps to gain a winning advantage.

These results for athletes also have implications for everyone. Sanctioned napping on the job can keep you focused and alert. It can provide superior decision-making ability that is crucial to your success, and it can do it in a way that stimulants can't. We think it's high time for employers to realize that giving permission for napping on the job can be highly beneficial to their employees and to their business.

Progress is being made. Dr. William Anthony, author of *The Art of Napping at Work* (1999) did an informal Internet survey of one thousand randomly selected people. Over 70 percent of this group indicated that they fell asleep at work. Some companies are taking this message to heart and allowing napping at work. They know that employees often miss work because of fatigue. Sanctioned napping reduces absenteeism and increases productivity and employee retention. It can also improve safety.

The US trucking and rail industries have instituted sanctioned napping policies. Hospitals are looking into it, and in some Asian companies a nap is required on every shift.

Companies allow coffee breaks and cigarette breaks, so why should a nap break be any different? Sleep researcher Sara Mednick compared the effects of a sixty- to ninety-minute nap with 200 mg of caffeine and a placebo. Her conclusion: "Overall, a daytime nap generally improved performance across three different learning paradigms, while caffeine impaired (or at least did not benefit) performance."[21]

Undoubtedly, napping is helpful for boosting our cognitive and physical abilities. However, let's not lose sight of the bigger problem. As Dr. David F. Dinges, a sleep researcher at the Perelman School of Medicine, notes, "Naps are a short-term fix, offering only temporary boosts in mental acuity. They cannot replace adequate recovery sleep over many days."

Do You Need a Nap?

Do you conk out at the movies or during a daytime flight? When you lie down in bed at night, are you out within five minutes?

Falling asleep the minute you enter a dark or dull environment, particularly if it's during daylight hours, is one of the hallmarks of sleep deprivation. By contrast, if you're getting *enough* sleep, you should be fairly peppy and alert during the day. It is daytime, after all.

But if you fall asleep on the train or while waiting for a meeting to begin, then sanctioned napping on the job may be just the cure you need. Although it sounds contrary to everything we've been led to believe about jobs, permitted napping while at work is actually a very good idea. It can bring you back to a peak level of performance in a relatively short amount of time. You don't need to descend into the deepest slow wave sleep to get this benefit. In fact, short naps less than thirty minutes long are often quite restorative, and they also produce the least sleep inertia or grogginess upon awakening.

CHAPTER EIGHTEEN

SLEEP HABITS OF HIGHLY SUCCESSFUL PEOPLE

Tonight, late, when I'm still not done with the day but must comply
with sleep, I can whisper, "There was done a little good today.
Today I changed myself and the world, just a little.
And yes, I loved." Most days, that is enough.

—Mary Anne Radmacher, *Live Boldly* (2008)

"Just tell me what I can do."

"Well, Jim, we have a lot of advice that—"

"Give me the most important things."

"Do you have a couple of hours?"

I was on the phone with a patient who wanted guidance on how sleep
might improve his success in the sales business.

"Can you boil it down to thirty minutes?"

"I'm not sure that would be—"

"I've got a notepad, Doc. Let's cover the territory."

This is the fast-paced approach of some businesspeople. So in the next few pages, we'll summarize what I told my patient. If you follow these suggestions, you'll undoubtedly wind up doing what he did—improving sleep habits and boosting overall performance on and off the job.

Sleep hygiene is an extremely important concept, and understanding the rationale behind it will help you get better sleep. Unfortunately, the term itself is somewhat misleading and untoward. It means *sleep practices and habits, particularly those relating to environmental and behavioral factors.* The term arose in a bygone era when lower standards of sanitation were commonplace. It originally referred to the literal cleanliness of the sleeping environment, especially as it related to bedbugs. Nineteenth-century beds had posts anchored in pots of oil to prevent insects from crawling up into the bed. Cleaning floors and rugs was difficult prior to the invention of power vacuum cleaners. Contagious diseases and other contaminants were more prevalent and problematic in the sleep environment.

Fortunately, most of us don't have to contend with sanitation to such a degree, and as a result the meaning of the term has evolved to reflect modern hindrances to healthy sleep. In contemporary usage sleep hygiene refers to all the practices and habits that are important for consistent, quality sleep and waking alertness. Good sleep hygiene can help you achieve the restful sleep required for optimum functioning. It encompasses the comfort and selection of bedding, room temperature, light and noise regulation, bedroom environment, regular bedtimes, eating, and exercising.

Attention to sleep hygiene is the first thing to look at when people have trouble sleeping. Some of these rules should be obvious, while others are more subtle. For example, the use of caffeine can have a negative effect on sleep. Surely everyone knows this, and yet many still believe that they're immune to this rule. A clock on the bedside table is a more subtle distraction, and the reason it is a deterrent to sleep may surprise you.

The following tips and recommendations are for normal sleepers, that is, people who don't suffer from insomnia. People with insomnia are treated differently (see Chapter 13. Insomnia is defined as the inability to fall asleep or stay asleep long enough.[1] For normal sleepers (that is, noninsomniacs), the main issue is trying to get them to change their behavior to take sleep seriously and get a sufficient amount of sleep on a consistent basis.

Most individuals who are having difficulty sleeping are well versed in the following recommendations, especially given the ubiquity of articles about proper sleep hygiene. Yet, it is important to keep in mind that knowing the rules and following the rules may be two different things. If you really intend to get your sleep back on track, you need to be willing to make some changes to your daily routines. These changes may be uncomfortable or irksome, especially at first, but you'll get used to them and you'll likely decide that they're worth the benefits of improved health, mood, and productivity. It's also important to realize how easy it is to underestimate or overestimate your own habits. Individual estimations of how much coffee you drink or how much TV you watch before bed, for example, can seem subjective. What doesn't feel like a lot of coffee to one person could in fact be a major culprit in his or her sleep troubles.[2] It's important to take an honest look at your own habits in order to make effective changes.

TIP #1: PRIORITIZE AND RESPECT SLEEP

Sleep should be managed as thoughtfully and deliberately as we manage our daytime schedules and activities. On this score, it's essential to be proactive about sleep needs, even if it means adding it to our to-do lists. We need to prioritize arranging our schedules to accommodate our optimal individual sleep requirements, devoting time and attention to our sleep needs just as we attend to daytime needs such as diet and fitness.

An enlightened mind-set concerning the biological need for sleep includes this fundamental principle:

WE DO NOT NEED TO MAKE APOLOGIES FOR REQUIRING
UNINTERRUPTED SLEEP OR NAPS, REGARDLESS OF THE TIME
OF DAY OR NIGHT, ANY MORE THAN WE NEED TO APOLOGIZE
FOR EATING OUR VEGETABLES OR GETTING EXERCISE.

Ideally, this mind-set will inform our interactions with others as well. It is reasonable to expect that family members, coworkers, and friends will respect our sleep needs and be respectful of variations in individual sleep requirements. It's also reasonable to expect others not to discredit the need for sleep or the person who needs it.

A close friend of David's is an excellent and compassionate psychiatrist. He tells every new patient about the rules that guide working with him. One rule that he is adamant about is that if the patient is going to have an emotional crisis, they must do so before 10:00 p.m. He considers sleep so important for his ability to help others that he protects it above all else. If the crisis is before 10:00 p.m., he will talk with them. If after 10:00 p.m., they must call 911. This demonstrates his understanding of the benefits of sleep, and it also models for his patients their own need to protect themselves.

Shifting toward this pro-sleep mind-set is how we begin to accommodate sleep at home, at school, and in the workplace. Go ahead and hang up DO NOT DISTURB signs, turn off your phone, and communicate the expectation that, like Napoleon, you won't tolerate being interrupted while you're sleeping.

Sleep is the new sex. People want it, need it, can't get enough of it.

—ARTHUR J. SPIELMAN, associate director of the Center for Sleep
Disorders Medicine and Research at New York Methodist Hospital

TIP #2: DETERMINE YOUR SLEEP NEEDS

Determining individual sleep needs can be tricky. Most of us tend to underestimate how much sleep we actually need, while others may overestimate that need. For example, many patients tell us they need eight hours of sleep every night to function optimally during the day. Yet on inquiry, they never get more than six hours of sleep and they're functioning well nevertheless. The general rule of thumb is the following.

> YOU NEED AS MUCH SLEEP AS IT TAKES TO ALLOW
> YOU TO FEEL ALERT DURING THE DAY.

Therein lies the rub. We tend to cover up sleepiness with caffeine and activity, which makes it difficult to determine whether we're actually functioning well or merely masking sleepiness. Dr. David F. Dinges and colleagues at the Perelman School of Medicine at the University of Pennsylvania have demonstrated that with chronic sleep restriction, people can't easily introspect their level of daytime sleepiness. The implication of this finding is that it is important to look for objective measures of sleepiness and not rely solely on your own estimation. For example, if you have no difficulty maintaining alertness while driving, do not fall asleep during sedentary activities such as reading or watching TV, and particularly if you awaken easily and spontaneously in the morning, you're probably getting an adequate amount of sleep. On the other hand, if any of these activities poses a problem, you may need to increase your sleep time. We believe it is important to point out here that sleep time alone may not be sufficient. An adequate sleep time with poor sleep quality can also leave you impaired during the day.

TIP #3: SET A BEDTIME (A WINDOW IS FINE)

If you're generally a good sleeper, once you've decided on your individual sleep need, it's important to set a bedtime to ensure you get sufficient sleep on a daily basis. With that being said, instead of an exact bedtime, we recommend a "bedtime window" that has a little latitude in either direction and is more real-world friendly. Obviously, if you're feeling especially exhausted, go to bed earlier than normal. If you're stuck at a business dinner that's running late, stressing about being out past your bedtime can cause problems in and of itself.

What is the best way to determine your individual bedtime? A normal *sleep latency* (the time it takes to fall asleep) should be about fifteen to twenty minutes. Simply add the length of time it takes you to fall asleep to your sleep need and calculate according to your wake-up time. For example, if your sleep need is eight hours, you have a normal sleep latency, and you wish to be up by 6:45 a.m., then you'll have to be in bed by about 10:25 p.m., which means starting your sleep routine even earlier. Sometimes it can take several days, or weeks, to calibrate your optimal individual sleep schedule. Incrementally increasing your sleep every night by as little as half an hour, or even fifteen minutes, can immediately and considerably improve the way you feel and function during the day.

TIP #4: BE PROTECTIVE OF YOUR SLEEP

It's an established fact that modern culture and technology are diametrically opposed to sleep sufficiency.[3] Resist the temptation to stay up watching late-night talk shows and surfing the Internet. They're not worth cutting into precious time that you could spend getting the sleep you need in order to optimize your level of functioning and quality of life. You must be as regular as you can with your sleep cycle to reap the optimum benefits of sleep. To this end, some people wisely set an alarm clock for *bedtime* rather than wake time.

TIP #5: SCHEDULE SLEEP

While most of us who are parents are pretty good at adhering to consistency for a child's bedtime (knowing full well the repercussions of failing to do so), we're more likely to disregard sleep consistency for ourselves. Variable bedtimes and wake-up times throughout the week can produce jet lag–like symptoms of fatigue, insomnia, and poor mood. Adults experience the same problems as young children when they have variable sleep schedules, including an inability to focus, irritability, and emotional problems.

A regular schedule, including consistent bedtime and wake time, is an important hygiene rule. While the body likes routine and regularity, we feel that wake time is the more important of the two. Going to bed at roughly the same time each night but not falling asleep for hours will lead to other forms of insomnia. Don't go to bed at ten o'clock just because your spouse goes to bed at that time or because ten seems like the time you should be in bed. Many people say to us, "I have to be up at seven in the morning and I need nine hours of sleep. I go to bed at ten so I'll get my nine hours." However, if it takes three hours to fall asleep, that person is actually getting only six hours of sleep. More important questions are: Do you feel sleepy at ten? Do you have trouble waking at seven? If you go to bed too early and have trouble falling asleep, you'll get frustrated and angry, your mind will begin to race, and you'll start to associate your bed and bedroom with wakefulness, not sleep. If it commonly takes several hours to fall asleep, you'll create an expectation that sleep will not occur. Like Pavlov's bell, the bed will make you more alert and even less likely to sleep. The bed is now a stimulus to wakefulness.[4] For good sleepers, by contrast, the bed and bedroom are a stimulus to sleep, and sleep is desired and looked forward to.

Your wake time is also more important because being awakened is a much stronger stimulus than falling asleep, and morning light tends to reset your biological clock. This is particularly true if you have difficulty waking up and require an alarm clock each morning. We aren't big fans of snooze alarms because hitting them is associated with thinking, *Ah! ten more minutes of blissful sleep*, rather than motivating you to get up. We instruct our patients to get out of bed reflexively once they hear the alarm. Waking up abruptly in the morning and getting exposed to light will help reset your internal clock. Exposure to morning bright light helps people fall asleep more easily in the evening hours.[5]

> Maintain a similar sleep schedule. This is really the number-one issue. When a person stays roughly on the same schedule, sleep drive is higher and the circadian rhythm is on track.
>
> —DR. MICHAEL BREUS, sleep scientist

TIP #6: ESTABLISH A PRESLEEP RITUAL

Many people abruptly drop into bed exhausted after a hectic day—but we advocate that you avoid doing that and, instead, implement an end-of-day routine. Such a bedtime routine or presleep ritual is crucial to train your body and mind to disengage and go into sleep mode. You would begin by winding down and relaxing prior to bedtime. Forty-five minutes to an hour is optimal, with half an hour being the minimum time you want to spend on this routine. For many of our patients who are having a difficult time falling asleep, the presleep routine includes soaking in a hot bath about forty-five minutes before bedtime. This can become more of a ritual by adding lavender oils, candles, and playing relaxing music. In addition to relaxation, these baths also provide a physiological enhancement: the lowering of body temperature that occurs upon leaving a warm bath is sleep inducing.

Ideally, your bedtime routine will generally follow the same steps in the same order each night, gradually bringing you closer to your bedroom. Once it's ingrained, your presleep ritual will become second nature. It will even be reproducible when you are traveling or sleeping in unfamiliar surroundings, enabling you to fall asleep more easily.

If you have children, you know the importance of a bedtime routine. For many youngsters, however, bedtime and going to sleep is like a time-out. After all, they're losing parental attention and access to their toys and electronics. The most effective bedtime routines for children are short and sweet and last about twenty to thirty minutes. It should be a clear indication to the child that it is time for bed. It should include some pleasant activity such as reading a book or cuddle time. This pleasant component is important because the child will look forward to bedtime rather than dreading it or seeing it as a punishment.

The reasoning behind a pleasant bedtime ritual for kids is easy to understand, but let's remember that we grown-ups deserve a similarly pleasant routine.

Our lives are often so busy that it may not be possible to accomplish all in a day that we would like. We try to press a little more time out of the day at the expense of our sleep. A good bedtime ritual can make sleep something to look forward to and can prevent unreasonable delay. On both a conscious and subconscious level, the ritual is telling the mind and body that sleep is important and pleasant, and in this way it begins the physiological changes necessary for sleep to occur. We consider the presleep ritual as encompassing all of the things that you actually do in a consistent manner each night to prepare for sleep. For example, putting on pj's, brushing teeth, brushing hair, and getting in bed. This is much different from, for example, putting on pj's, getting in bed, reading emails, responding as needed, discussing finances with your bed partner, and reading the report that you'll present tomorrow. The key idea is that the ritual is geared to winding down and promoting sleep rather than squeezing in a few more minutes of work. You might find it helpful to think of the forty-five minutes set aside for your presleep ritual as an interlude during which your mind will be shifting away from the stresses of the day. This is your "let it go" time. You'll have plenty of opportunity to worry during the day. Don't do it during this presleep interval. Instead, get in the elevator and press the button for S: "Subbasement, please." Make all stops on the way down to deep, restful sleep.

Music to Help You Fall Asleep

The right type of music can help some people fall asleep. As clinicians, we have found that the most effective type of music is soft and slow, around sixty beats per minute, with no words and no wide variations in tempo or style. A 2015 meta-analysis by K. V. Jespersen and colleagues aimed at assessing the effects of listening to music on insomnia in adults came to a similar conclusion. Reviewing a total of six studies comprising 314 study subjects, the meta-analysis examined the effect of listening to prerecorded music daily before sleep, for twenty-five to sixty minutes, for a period of three days to five weeks. Music was found to be a safe, nonpharmacological intervention that's easy to administer and may be effective for improving subjective sleep quality in adults with insomnia symptoms. The authors concluded that additional research is needed to establish the effect of listening to music on other aspects of sleep.

TIP #7: CALM YOUR MIND

Put aside any work, arguments, or complicated decisions as bedtime approaches. It may take some time to turn off the emotional and intellectual noise of the day. One of the most common complaints we hear from patients is, "My mind races at night when I try to fall asleep." To help decrease ruminating at night about your obligations or worries, keep a to-do list that includes a "things to worry about" list—some may refer to this as a worry journal. Around dinnertime you can bring it up to date, add new items, and make new entries—but then leave it for the day and never review it or revisit it close to bedtime. And whatever you do, never *ever* bring your to-do list or worry journal into your bedroom! Keep it outside the room, at least for symbolic purposes. However, we do advocate keeping pen and paper at your bedside in the event you come up with an idea, solution, song lyrics, or plot for a novel in the middle of the night or upon awakening.

TIP #8: AVOID THE CLOCK

Almost every list of sleep hygiene rules will include not having a clock on a bedside table. This may seem trivial, but in fact the bedside clock is a very powerful stimulus to arousal. The moment your eye looks at the clock, you calculate two numbers: how long you have been there and how much time you have left. Both of those numbers can be anxiety provoking. But there is actually a more profound reason why the clock on the bedside table is a bad idea. Even good sleepers awaken five to ten or more times each night. We are often unaware of this awakening because sleep has amnestic properties. That is, you forget what happens right before you fall asleep. If you immediately go back to sleep, you'll forget that you ever awakened and it will seem as if you slept without awakening. If there is a clock by your bedside, your eye may catch the clock on one of these normal arousals, causing apprehension and changing a fifteen-second arousal into a thirty-minute awakening. It's a good idea to set the alarm so that you're certain you will get up in the morning, but turn the face of the clock away from you so that you don't see the time during the night. God help you if you have a grandfather clock that chimes every quarter hour during the night. Once your sleep schedule is normalized and you're getting sufficient sleep, you may even find that you can get by just fine *without* having a clock in the room. And that, friend, is a sure sign that you're becoming a super sleeper.

TIP #9: NO ELECTRONICS IN THE BEDROOM

Most sleep hygiene lists say that there should not be a television in the bedroom. There are many reasons for this. More nighttime television means less sleep for many Americans. Obviously, if you're watching television and engaged in the program, it's very difficult to fall asleep. Also, by watching television in bed the stimulus value (the strength of a stimulus to elicit a response) of the bed for sleep is completely lost. You now begin associating the bed with a great place to watch Jimmy Kimmel.

Secondly, many people will leave the television on all night. We're told that they do this because their mind is so active that they need a distraction, and a television playing in the background will allow them to fall asleep. However, keeping the television on all night will actually disrupt sleep. The light levels on televisions change dramatically with bright and dark flickers, and the volume can also change substantially. In addition, the contents of the audio can vary from light music to loud screams. We believe taking the television out of the bedroom (and all other screens and chargers) is a good idea.

If it's a good idea for you, it's an even better idea for your children. In the United States, an estimated 20 percent of infants and toddlers less than two years old have a television in their bedroom. Studies have shown that children sleeping with a TV in the room experience shorter sleep durations.[6] Remember that the television isn't designed to put children to sleep but to attract their attention, and electronics emit short wavelengths, the blue light that is activating to children and adults.

David's story illustrates this point: I recently saw a four-year-old who couldn't get to sleep or stay asleep. The family all slept in the same room. I discussed the need for the television to be off at night but was met with a great deal of resistance from the parents. Both parents reported that they kept the television on all night as this was the only way they could sleep. For the sake of their child, they said that they would try a week without the television on at night. I was doubtful that this child's sleep would improve, feeling that the parents could not go a week without their electronic crutch. To my pleasant surprise, when I saw them back they reported that the child's sleep had improved substantially. Both parents were actually grinning and stated that their sleep had also improved. Sometimes little changes can make a big difference.

TIP #10: NO ALL-NIGHT RADIO OR MUSIC

We also see many patients who keep some form of music on all night and then complain that they can't sleep. This seems to be more common with young people. As with those who keep the television on, the common response when we question people about this habit is that it helps distract their active minds. A totally quiet room allows their minds too much room to wander, and they find it difficult to shut thoughts down for the night. Remember that insomnia is a disorder of thinkers. During the day an active mind is a good thing and it can serve you well. But at night it can be a problem. Using the radio, however, is a poor solution.

For many of the same reasons that we recommend keeping televisions off in the bedroom at night, we also recommend keeping music off at night. The radio can switch rapidly from music to voices and the volume can vary. If you do fall asleep and there's a sudden change in the volume or style of sound, the transition can awaken you or at least fragment your sleep. Remember that natural awakenings occur several times each night (see the hypnogram on page 17). If the room is dark and quiet, there's a good chance you'll return to sleep very quickly. However, if you awaken and hear a particularly good song, you may have enough cognitive arousal to delay a return to sleep. The type of music is also important. We see many young people who think there's no problem with listening to loud rock or aggressive music as they're making an effort to sleep, yet they can't understand why they're having sleep problems.

It's true that if music isn't played continuously throughout the night and is of the right variety, it may help some people fall asleep. Several studies do support using music for sleep induction. Researchers including Professor Hui-Ling Lai at Tzu Chi University, Taiwan, have shown that forty-five minutes of relaxing music before bedtime can make for a restful night. Taiwanese researchers found that soft, slow music caused physical changes that aided restful sleep, including lower heart and respiratory rates. The researchers also found that people listening to music in their study reported a 35 percent improvement in sleep quality, including better and longer nighttime sleep with less dysfunction during the following day. Numerous studies demonstrate that music has a statistically significant sleep-promoting effect,[7] which may explain and substantiate the almost universal and timeless tradition of lullabies.

TIP #11: LIMIT BEDTIME READING

Most sleep hygiene lists also recommend that you don't read in bed. The strictest approach is that the bed should be reserved for sleep and sex and, other than that, you shouldn't be in the bed. We bend the reading rule to some degree. Many people find that reading for a few minutes helps distract their active minds, allows them to get drowsy, and helps them fall asleep. Numerous patients have told us that they open a book on the couch and actually fall asleep while reading. However, getting up and walking to the bedroom may be enough physical activity to make it more difficult to fall asleep. For this reason, we do allow reading in the bedroom for a few minutes prior to sleep onset, but this needs to be individualized. If space permits, it's recommended that a comfortable chair in the room is better for reading and for transitioning into the bed for sleep.

Be cautious about reading before bed, though. Many people get so caught up in the story that they stay up for hours so that they can find out what will happen next. For this reason, we suggest reading material that isn't particularly suspenseful, such as nonengaging nonfiction. Some find that the more mindless the better, such as thumbing through catalogues. Unfortunately, John F. Kennedy didn't know about this rule, read James Bond novels before bed, and suffered from insomnia.[8]

We also prohibit doing work that involves reading at bedtime. However, if you're one of those people who can fall asleep while reading, relax the rule. If reading keeps you up, then limit your reading to outside the bedroom. It also helps to use the lowest wattage lightbulb to read—15 watts is preferable.

In our opinion, the Energy Independence and Security Act of 2007, which phases out incandescent bulbs in favor of fluorescent ones, is a grave mistake. Fluorescent lights may provide some small energy savings, but we expect the toll in disrupted sleep as a result of increased exposure to blue wavelengths, which are present in higher amounts in these new bulbs, to be devastating.

TIP #12: USE THE BED ONLY FOR SLEEP AND SEX

While we bend the rules a little by allowing reading, the maxim "the bed is for sleep or sex" is generally a good one. The point is, we want the bed and the bedroom to maintain a stimulus value for sleep as much as possible. When you do things other than sleep in the bed, that stimulus value is diluted or lost entirely. The examples of reading, television, and music are fairly subtle. More extreme examples can become serious problems. We once saw a couple who basically lived in their bed and bedroom. They would spend the entire evening, from five o'clock on, in bed, playing games with their children, watching television, reading the newspaper, and even eating dinner in bed. The bedroom had lost any special significance for sleep, and both of them had sleep problems.

Amber Glasses

One of the newest high-tech methods of getting better sleep is based on the recent discovery that blue wavelengths of light are especially disruptive to sleep architecture. Dr. Charles Czeisler of Harvard Medical School demonstrated as early as 1981 that sunlight keeps our internal clock running smoothly. The widespread prevalence of computer screens, cell phones, and new so-called energy-efficient bulbs is disrupting normal sleep. These devices all emit blue wavelength light, the kind that interferes with melatonin production more than light of other colors.

We have noted several times in this book that light has a powerful effect on sleep, particularly blue wavelength light. In order to entrain to the twenty-four-hour day, we must reset our clocks every morning. To do this we require light. The image-producing cells in the retina are called rods and cones, but surprisingly, these rods and cones are *not* required to condition us to the circadian rhythms. Early work by Russell Foster and others revealed that mice that didn't have rods or cones could still be entrained to the light-dark cycle.[9] This surprising fact led to the discovery of a novel retinal ganglion cell in humans that does not produce an image; instead, it responds to blue wavelengths by firing directly from the eye into the suprachiasmatic nucleus (SCN), a tiny region located in the hypothalamus. The SCN is the main circadian oscillator (clock), and SCN nerve impulses suppress melatonin. Even if a person is totally blind, provided this eye-to-SCN pathway is intact, they'll still stay in rhythm with the light-dark cycle.[10] This pathway also uses a special photosensitive chemical called melanopsin,[11] a photopigment that is activated by light between 420 and 440 nm. This is blue light.[12] Put more simply, special ganglion cells in the retina don't produce images but instead send impulses directly to the master clock. These cells are most highly activated by blue light, and this explains why blue wavelengths are capable of shifting circadian rhythms, depending on when the organism is exposed to this light.[13]

Amber-colored glasses to the rescue? Free software programs such as f.lux can change the color spectrum of your computer. Using such a program at night is a good idea since it automatically gives your screen a sleep-enhancing red shift. The advantage of such a color change is that you'll be exposed to less blue light at night. But because there are so many other sources of blue light in our environment, it's also a good idea to use amber-colored glasses, which block the blue wavelengths that act to keep people awake by interfering with melatonin production and through other physiological pathways. Bottom line: the use of yellow lenses will block light in the blue spectrum and limit the ability of the SCN cells to disrupt natural circadian rhythms.

TIP #13: DON'T MAKE THE BEDROOM AN OFFICE

If space permits, avoid using the bedroom as an office, multipurpose room, or storage place for unfolded laundry and stacks of junk mail. If space does not permit, put as much of it away at the close of the day as possible. Shut down, power off, and move paperwork out of sight. Keep the bedroom as clutter-free as possible.

TIP #14: STOP *TRYING* TO SLEEP

This is a subtle point and one that is somewhat difficult to explain. We hear people say, "I go to bed and try to sleep." That one little sentence already suggests a problem. *Try* is an arousing word. If we say, "Try to lift your desk," you'll instantly feel your muscles tense as you activate your body for physical exertion. If you go to bed and try to sleep, you've already lost the battle. You'll begin to feel your muscles tense, your respiratory rate quicken, and perhaps even your heart rate increase. Sleep needs to be allowed—it can't be forced. You have to let it overtake you. You have to give in to it, which is very difficult for many people.

Letting go is particularly hard for people who like a great deal of control in their lives. For example, we saw a patient who said that he controlled everything in his life and felt that he could control his sleep similarly. But it doesn't quite work like that. If you have to try to sleep, something is already wrong. This is why a rule for insomniacs says, Go to bed only when you're sleepy, not just because it is ten o'clock. If your mind is active at bedtime and you need a distraction to allow sleep to overtake you, activity such as meditation, self-hypnosis, progressive muscle relaxation, or even the proverbial counting sheep can help.[14] These techniques take advantage of the active mind but use it to the sleeper's advantage.

TIP #15: AVOID NIGHTCAPS

Alcohol is often referred to as a nightcap, implying that it can be used at bedtime as a sleep aid. As we all know, alcohol is an interesting drug. However, it's unsettling how many people rely on alcohol as a primary means of getting to sleep. It's true that alcohol is one of the few substances that actually increases stage 3 NREM sleep. In addition, it may help people fall asleep more quickly. However, alcohol isn't effective at producing quality sleep. The ability of alcohol to increase deep sleep and shorten sleep onset only works with infrequent or short-term use. That is, after a day or two of using alcohol to help you sleep, you will lose these few benefits. Even with acute use, the benefits of alcohol are limited to the first two to three hours of the night. As alcohol is metabolized, it will actively wake you up. In addition, alcohol selectively decreases muscle tone in the upper airway. This is why some people don't snore unless they consume alcohol. Alcohol can create sleep apnea in a person who normally doesn't have obstructed breathing during sleep. In short, alcohol is not a good short-term or long-term solution for sleep problems. We are primarily concerned with the use of alcohol in the three hours prior to bedtime. A glass of wine at dinner will probably not have a negative effect on sleep. However, a few drinks right before bedtime can certainly create significant problems. If you are having trouble sleeping, do not resort to alcohol as a solution.

Chronotypes

What's your diurnal preference? In other words, are you a morning or evening person? Larks feel better and more alert in the mornings; owls prefer evenings. Your tendency either way (or somewhere in the middle) is for the large part genetically determined (a gene called PER3, to be exact). In 1998, researchers at the University of Surrey published results of a study undertaken to test the validity of Benjamin Franklin's maxim "Early to bed and early to rise makes a man healthy, wealthy, and wise." The study of 1,229 men and women found that night owls had larger mean incomes and were better off financially, with "a comfortable home, a nonmanual job, and access to a car." No health or cognitive advantages were noted between the two groups. The study's findings failed to support Franklin's claim; indeed, being late to bed and late to rise doesn't seem to negatively impact socioeconomic, cognitive, or health status. In fact, another study of 420 people published in 1999 by Roberts and Kyllonen reported higher intelligence scores in owls.

Famous larks include George H. W. Bush, George W. Bush, Rachel Ray, Tim Cook, Condoleezza Rice, Howard Schultz, Ernest Hemingway, Benjamin Franklin, and John Grisham.

Famous night owls include Barack Obama, Charles Darwin, Marissa Mayer, Hillary Clinton, Adolf Hitler, Winston Churchill, James Joyce, Fran Lebowitz, Keith Richards, Honoré de Balzac, and Elvis Presley.

Knowing how much of a lark or an owl you are might improve your sleep health and overall quality of life. Obviously, work schedules are a huge consideration. Owls prefer go to work later and stay later, to be self-employed, and to work from home. Both larks and owls need to be more strategic about light exposure: they should make a point of getting light upon awakening and cutting out blue light close to bedtime. Mixing owls and larks in a relationship can lead to trouble, which raises the question, *Can you switch from being a night to a morning person?* Some people have done so successfully for various reasons, and the process is most likely a gradual one with a lot of motivation needed. Our body clocks tend to fluctuate over a lifetime. Small children wake early, while teens wake late. The elderly tend to wake early, too.

Says David: Anecdotally, I can tell you from my experience that owls tend to marry larks. Sometimes the differences become larger as the relationship continues. For example, maybe the owl started staying up later to let his spouse fall asleep before he began snoring. Or perhaps the lark developed to get up with the children. Regardless of why it happens, it can be difficult to change. Owls often like the solitude of late night to focus on thoughts or projects without interruption. I've been asked to help change the clocks of some owls, and it's often easier to find jobs that allow owls to be who they are. Larks have rarely asked for help in changing their sleep habits. Larks make poor shift workers. As a proud owl, I'll note that larks tend to be self-righteous, feeling they're morally better than us. The larks are always trying to impose larkishness on the rest of us. Owls never seem to impose their schedule on others.

As we've already noted, sleep has to be allowed; it can't be forced, yet it is often difficult to allow sleep to overtake you. Engaging in activities such as counting sheep, self-hypnosis, meditation, or deep breathing exercises may actually help distract some people from the fact that they're trying to fall asleep. This kind of helpful distraction may set the stage to focus the mind *away* from trying to sleep, ultimately allowing the physiology of sleep to lull you into slumberland. Such an approach and a bedtime routine are two of the most powerful ways that we know to help you sleep for success.

For most people, following the sleep hygiene rules listed above will work wonders to change their sleep patterns from troublesome to terrific. These suggestions have worked for many other people and they are likely to be the foundation for your good sleep, too. If we could sit down with you and ask about your particular sleep habits, chances are that we would wind up our interview by giving you a printed list of the rules we have enumerated above. We would ask you to try to implement them to the best of your ability for three weeks. Once these rules become sleep habits, you're on your way to better, more successful sleep.

If you've come this far in the book, you're ready to make those changes! We've seen countless people do it, with good results. We're here to tell you that in all likelihood you can do it, too.

CHAPTER NINETEEN

SLEEPING YOUR WAY TO THE TOP

Let her sleep, for when she wakes, she will move mountains.

—Napoleon Bonaparte

———

In conclusion, Terry would like to tell you a true story that illustrates the key thesis of this book. A good-natured older woman brought her grown daughter into the clinic one day. Her daughter was divorced and living at her mother's home with her children. The woman said she could hear her daughter snoring loudly at night, loud enough to wake the other members of the household.

The daughter was in her early forties, a surly, if not angry, overweight woman who wanted nothing to do with a sleep study. She was verbally abusive to her mother at the appointment. She didn't agree with her mother's concerns about her sleep, her snoring, her weight gain, or her moodiness.

At her mother's insistence, and after much cajoling, the daughter was tested and found to have severe sleep apnea and was promptly treated with CPAP. After all was said and done, the mother came back to the clinic one afternoon with goodies for the staff, and I'll never forget her words.

"Thank you . . . for giving me back my daughter."

She described how unhappy her daughter had been prior to diagnosis, how she yelled at her kids all the time and was in a bad mood from the moment she woke up to the moment she went to bed. With CPAP treatment, her daughter was happier, easygoing, didn't complain about her job, and seemed to be back to her good-natured self.

That's the kind of dramatic change that sufficient sleep can produce. Think of her family members, her employer, her colleagues, her quality of life, and the quality of life for those around her. If you don't think diagnosis and treatment of sleep disorders can be life changing, remember this woman.

Throughout this treatise we've been telling you about the value of sleep, and about the concomitant dangers of sleep deprivation. You now know, for example, that losing sleep can weaken your immune system, worsen your mood, make it more difficult for others to read your emotional state, and impair your ability to perform at your best. The flip side is equally true. Regularly getting the sleep you need will quicken your reflexes, boost your athletic prowess, make it easier for you to lead others, brighten your mood, raise your emotional intelligence, and sharpen your memory. If you're a musician, it will improve your performance. If you're a businessperson, it will help you deal more effectively with customers. The list goes on and on, and this is just the tip of the iceberg about how sleep can improve your game, whatever it happens to be. For heaven's sake, sufficient sleep even makes you look better.

We hope you've been inspired to prioritize and protect sleep. We don't want you to become paranoid, but you know that you're living in a culture that devalues this precious biological commodity. You saw how blue wavelength light interferes with sleep, and how you can fight the onslaught of sleep-disruptive technology with good sleep hygiene and a mind-set that values sleep.

This volume, we daresay, might even be your secret weapon. The message it announces, together with the specific sleep strategies it describes, is similar to a modern philosophy. In the same way that Spinoza, Nietzsche, and Sartre show you how to view life and experience it to the fullest, we offer you a philosophy, too. Only our philosophy is rooted in scientific research. Ours is a philosophy of the mind, a true practical psychology. We offer our philosophy to you with the conviction that our way of thinking about sleep can produce profound changes for the better in anyone who heeds its message.

Despite the prolific propaganda advocating an opposite point of view, sufficient sleep is actually the dirty little secret of highly successful people. Simply put, sleep can make or break you. Not only are we collectively guilty of ignoring sleep, we've been guilty of spurning sleep, probably the singular most destructive thing we could voluntarily do to limit ourselves and our chances for success.

As clinicians, we see miraculous changes that happen every day when people obtain sufficient sleep. So we'll leave you with this simple but proven call to action. Through knowledge comes power. We trust that this little guidebook has empowered you—to learn more about sleep, to respect sleep, to manage sleep, and to reap the amazing and life-changing benefits that sufficient sleep can bestow. Go ahead and make sleep a personal value, a family value, and a workplace value. You'll feel better and do better in all of your endeavors. Then get the sleep you need. Put down the remote, turn off the phone, take a warm bath, climb into bed, read a chapter from this book, switch off the light, and let your journey begin: a journey into an unconscious realm that can change you for the better, a journey that will allow you to do more, achieve more, and produce more, since night after night you'll be sleeping your way to the top.

ACKNOWLEDGMENTS

It is with great pleasure that we acknowledge the many friends, researchers, and colleagues who have contributed immeasurably to our thinking on the subject of sleep over the past three decades. This volume draws on more than ten thousand pages of articles, scientific reports, and research studies conducted by some of the most eminent scholars in the field of sleep medicine. At the outset we would like to thank the librarians at the University of Texas Southwestern Medical School in Dallas, Randolph-Macon College, and Virginia Commonwealth University.

We should be deficient in graciousness as well as gratitude were we to close this section of our manuscript without mentioning those fellow researchers with whom we have had the pleasure of working over the years, not only during our education at the outset of our academic career, but also during the first years of clinical practice, when exciting new discoveries and interactions with patients caused the world of sleep science to come alive for us as never before. To this end we would like to particularly mention William Dement, Andrew Jamieson, and Christian Guilleminault. We would be thoughtless to neglect mentioning our deep appreciation for our mentors and associates John Herman, Howard Roffwarg, Milt Erman, Phillip Becker, Andrew Jamieson, Michael Sateia, and Teofilo Lee-Chiong. We are ever mindful of the many kindnesses of Judith Owens and Mary Carskadon.

Having now come to the end of our labors on this monologue, after more than two years of strenuous effort—which has not been without its rewards—it is only fitting that we thank the man who lit the way for us when the road was dark, our literary agent, Steve Harris, a visionary who not only saw the merits in our book even in its fledgling stages, but who also encouraged us not to give up when the going got tough. And it is not without regret that we now, upon publication of this book, part company with our industrious and dedicated co-writer William Cane, a tireless and inventive collaborator whose assistance allowed us to push further into the research than we had expected in the time allotted to us to complete this project. Thanks are due, also, to Andrea Au Levitt, senior editor at Reader's Digest Adult Trade Books, who gave us valuable feedback during the early stages of our work. At Sterling Publishing we are grateful for the careful review of our manuscript by Kirsten Colton, our copyeditor, and Kate Zimmermann, our editor. We also would like to thank the cadre of proofreaders, designers, and other artists and artisans without whose assistance this volume would have been an impossibility.

We would be remiss were we to neglect the sincere and ardent assistance we received from our associates, friends, and families, so it gives us true satisfaction to thank all who stood by our side while we devoted time to the completion of this volume. In particular, it is with heartfelt gratitude, immense appreciation, and infinite admiration that Terry would like to thank Dr. Naim Bashir, Dr. and Mrs. Demetrios Julius, David and Judith Moore, Dr. Gregg Korbon, Dr. Alexander Saloman, Robert Huff, Candace Johnson, Ed Grandi, Lynda and Roy Harrill, Avery Chenoweth, Jacqueline Edwards, Kate Fiddyment, Terra Ziporyn Snider, Dave Perry, Tim Leinbaugh, Randy Thompson, Mary Helen Uusimaki, Jasmine Wood, Ryan Trainer, Genevieve Piturro, David and Shannon Farley, Lewis T. Stoneburner, Fran Kizer, Baylor Belford, Lori Casto, Jaimie Murdock, Rhonda Hunt, Jenny Highlander, Robin Sevachko, Andrew Selfridge; and forever in loving memory of Harold P. Leinbaugh and Margaret Bickett. Terry would especially like to thank Den Cralle for his valuable input and unwavering support. David would like to thank his children, David, Christopher, and Will.

NOTES

1. Trumping Sleep

1. Sleep apnea is a disorder in which the airway is obstructed, leading to the sleeper becoming oxygen deprived and rising from deep to lighter stages of sleep. Most people who have sleep apnea do not know it.

2. George and Davis 2013.

3. There are at least two types of short sleepers: those with a genetic predisposition to need little sleep, and those with "a behavioral imposition" (Kushida 2004:509).

4. Gartner 2011.

5. Jones 2013 (discussing Gallup poll).

6. Rath and Harter 2010.

3. Sleep is *Not a Dirty Word*

1. Wiley and Formby 2001:24. Sleep deprivation affects a considerable number of people—up to 47 million American adults, or about one in five. According to the 2005 to 2008 National Health and Nutrition Examination Survey, more than one-third of individuals report sleeping less than seven hours per night during the week, and studies at the University of Chicago and Cornell University found that people who claimed to sleep seven to eight hours per night actually slept closer to six hours.

2. Salord et al 2015. *See also* Surani et al 2015 (sleep apnea associated with diabetes).

3. Alvarez and Ayas 2004.

4. Van Cauter et al 2005, and St-Onge 2013. Dr. Eve Van Cauter, sleep researcher and professor of medicine at the University of Chicago, notes that people take pride in not getting much sleep. However, she makes the interesting analogy to smoking, suggesting that twenty years from now not getting enough sleep will seem dangerous. Just as smoking (and drunk driving) became unpopular as the risks came to light, so will sleep deprivation.

5. Spiegel et al 2004. *See also* Spiegel et al 1999 (sleep debt harms carb metabolism and endocrine function).

4. Not Now, I'm Tired

1. See chapter 3, note 1.

2. Sleep deprivation can be acute or chronic in nature. Acute sleep deprivation refers to no sleep or a reeducation in the usual total sleep time, usually lasting one or two days. Chronic sleep deprivation exists when the individual routinely sleeps less than required for optimal functioning.

3. Eickhoff et al 2015.

4. Sallinen et al 2008.

5. Wehr 1992.

6. This data on the impossibility of making up sleep loss in just two nights helped us win a lawsuit where an individual fatally fell asleep while driving after trying to catch up on sleep over one weekend.

7. *See* Williamson and Feyer 2000 (sleep deprivation is like being inebriated).

8. Harvard Health Publications 2007.

9. Ma et al 2015 (meta-analysis of studies on sleep loss and the attending brain).

10. Van Dongen et al 2003 (people unaware of effects of sleep loss). *See also* Cohen et al 2010.

5. Sleep and Grow Rich

1. Ritter and Dijksterhuis 2014.

2. Cai et al 2009.

3. Wagner et al 2004.

4. Walker et al 2002.

5. *See* Barrett 2001.

6. Siegel et al 1998.

7. *See* Barrett 2001.

8. A. E. van Vogt is probably one of the most extreme examples of dream mining. He set an alarm clock to wake himself up every ninety minutes so that he could mine his dreams for story ideas (Platt 1980).

9. German researchers demonstrated this problem-solving aspect of dreams by having subjects perform a lengthy mathematical manipulation to get a desired result. Unknown to subjects, there was a hidden rule that facilitated finding the solution. Subjects were tested twelve hours apart, with one group sleeping and the other staying awake. The sleep group more than doubled the discovery of the hidden rule compared with the wake group (Wagner et al 2004).

10. It certainly was for Paul McCartney, who dreamed the song "Yesterday."

11. Jackson 2007:2.

12. It has been observed that modern art can produce extraordinary wealth for a select group of artists who have little talent except for exploiting the gullibility of critics (Wolfe 1975).

13. The half-asleep intervals immediately after awakening (hypnopompia) and prior to slumber (hypnagogia) are, similarly, times when the mind produces solutions and creative insights (Hale-Evans 2006:107–108).

14. Sheth, Janvelyan, and Kahn 2008.

15. Erlacher 2012.

16. Sio, Monaghan, and Ormerod 2013. *See also* Walker 2002.

6. Strange Bedfellows

1. There are 146.3 million working civilians in the United States (Bureau of Labor Statistics 2015), and 50 to 70 million of them chronically suffer from a sleep disorder (Colten and Altevogt 2006).

2. *See* Cohen et al 2010.

3. Colten and Altevogt 2006.

4. *See* Katz, Pront, and Lowry 2014 (employees who slept well experienced significantly more productivity).

5. Luckhaupt 2012.

6. Schor 1991.

7. Americans have added 160 hours yearly to their work and commute in the last thirty years. That is equivalent to an extra month of work and commute time. A 2002 estimate of global work hours from the Organization for Economic Co-Operation and Development Outlook found US workers working two hundred to four hundred more hours than workers in France, Norway, Sweden, Denmark, and Germany. There is worse news for working mothers, whose workload has increased by no less than 241 hours in a year.

8. *See* Kucharczyk, Morgan, and Hall 2012 (insomnia causes reduced productivity) and Katz, Pronk, and Lowry 2014 (insufficient sleep causes reduced productivity).

9. Sleep deprivation impairs attention, ingenuity, confidence, memory, leadership, and decision making. It leads to suboptimal decision making, particularly for decisions that rely on emotional processing. These decision-making deficits are not reversible with stimulants. So while a cup of coffee may provide a temporary increase in energy, the deleterious effects of sleep deprivation can be remedied only with sleep (Killgore, Grugle, and Balkin 2012).

Some examples of accidents attributed to sleep deprivation include:

1979—Three Mile Island meltdown (4:00 a.m.).

1984—Bhopal explosion (just after midnight).

1986—Chernobyl nuclear accident (1:26 a.m.).

1986—The *Challenger* space shuttle disaster.

1988—Peach Bottom Nuclear Reactor shutdown; workers were found sleeping on the job.

1989—*Exxon Valdez* oil spill (12:04 a.m.).

Humans get two hours of performance for each one hour of sleep. If there isn't enough sleep to cover performance, the brain finds a way of getting the sleep it needs. "It's almost as if the brain says, 'If you won't give me sleep, I'll sneak it in when you're not looking,'" said Navy captain Nick Davenport when discussing the *Challenger* disaster.

10. *See* Akerstedt et al 2002.

11. A 2012 poll commissioned by Central Queensland University and bedding manufacturer Sealy of more than thirteen thousand Australians revealed that 70 percent experienced reduced productivity at work because of a lack of sleep, and 38 percent admitted to dozing off on the job.

In 2012, Dr. Alexandra Michel of the University of Southern California's Marshall School of Business published the results of a nine-year study of investment bankers. Overworked, stressed out, and plagued with sleep deprivation, many of the study's participants were "a mess" by the fourth year, exhibiting overall declines in performance. Depression and substance abuse rates grew, while some were diagnosed with long-term health conditions such as Crohn's disease, psoriasis, rheumatoid arthritis, and thyroid disorders. Some had even developed explosive tempers. By the sixth year of the study, 40 percent of the participants decided to prioritize their health by limiting their work hours and paying more attention to sleep, diet, and exercise as a result of health and emotional problems.

12. *Merriam-Webster Collegiate Dictionary* (online edition) 2015.

13. *See* Benson 1975 (discussing importance of relaxing in American culture).

14. Kivimäki et al 2011.

15. Akerstedt et al 2002.

16. One large European study of over three thousand workers found that job stressors had a direct impact on sleep quality that was independent of hours worked or lifestyle factors. In one of the few studies looking at American workers, it was shown that in 1,700 full-time workers, job stress was again found to be a significant factor contributing to poor sleep quality. There were some interesting comments made in this study. Job stress can be broken down into several different independent factors, such as work overload and job control. The latter focuses on the degree of decision-making authority workers have over how they perform their jobs. The argument is that high demands and low control are risk factors for a variety of negative health-related outcomes, including poor sleep. The study suggests that having more decision latitude in a job is a protective factor in terms of sleep quality.

17. Sallinen et al 2008.

18. *See*, e.g., Lallukka 2014.

19. Steffen et al 2015.

20. Kling, McLeod, and Koehoorn 2010.

21. Kucharczyk, Morgan, and Hall 2012.

22. Luckhaupt 2012.

23. Huffington 2015.

7. Staying Power

1. Hubpages 2014.

2. *See* Montville 2007 (sleep helped Ruth play better).

3. Elliot 2014.

4. Ericsson, Krampe, and Tesch-Römer 1993 (Olympic athletes sleep close to eight hours and nap half an hour a day).

5. Tucker 2013.

6. Yoo et al 2007.

7. Leproult and Van Cauter 2011. *See also* Swerdloff and Wang 2011.

8. Muller et al 2005 (higher testosterone associated with better cognitive performance). *See also* Bremner 2010.

9. Spiegel, Leproult, and Van Cauter 1999.

10. *See* Fullagar et al 2015.

11. Kamdar et al 2004. *See also* Thun et al 2014 (sleep extension improves athletic performance).

12. Walker et al 2002.

13. *Id.*

14. Ericsson, Krampe, and Tesch-Römer 1993.

15. Fullagar et al 2015.

16. Poussel et al 2015. Another strategy that helped athletes was avoiding early-morning starts (Sargent et al 2014a; early-morning starts increase fatigue) and avoiding early-morning training (Sargent, Halson, and Roach 2014b; early-morning training not beneficial for world-class swimmers).

17. Mah et al 2011.

18. Kamdar et al 2004. *See also* Walker and Stickgold 2005 (athletic skill improves during sleep).

19. Juliff, Halson, and Peiffer 2015.

20. Hatfield 2007.

21. *See* Manfredini et al 1998.

8. If You've Got It, Flaunt It

1. Axelsson et al 2010:5.

2. Molloy 1996:98.

3. Rhodes 2006.

4. *See* Meskó, Paál, and Gábor 2012 (long-haired women perceived as more attractive).

5. Axelsson et al 2010:4.

6. Pfann et al 2006.

7. Madera and Hebl 2012.

8. Chervin et al 2013.

9. Oyetakin-White et al 2015.

10. There is "no reliable evidence to support the claim that these [topical] products have the same effects as prescription HGH, which is always given by injection" (Ratini

2014). The fragrance of essential oils, however, has been shown to help some people sleep better, which could help boost skin-friendly HGH. *See,* e.g., Sergeeva et al 2010 (scent of jasmine is as sleep inducing as prescription sleeping pills).

9. Sleeping with the Stars

1. Van Dongen et al 2003, and Jones 2011.

2. Belenky et al 2003.

3. Tate 2015, and Ascher-Walsh 2012.

4. Hall 2015.

5. Most short sleepers suffer from negative impacts on health or performance (Seystahl et al 2014).

6. Chang et al 2015 (light-emitting eReaders negatively affect sleep).

7. Bush 2013:504.

8. *Id.*

9. Manfred 2014.

10. *Id.*

10. You Are What You Sleep

1. Killgore et al 2007.

2. Fleischman 2004.

3. *See* Dinges et al 1997 (two nights of recovery needed). *See also* Lucassen et al 2014 (sleep-deprived obese people exhibit neurocognitive deficits that are partially reversed after makeup sleep).

4. Barnes, Gunia, and Wagner 2015.

5. *Id.*

6. Olsen, Pallesen, and Eid 2010 (moral reasoning diminished in sleep-deprived military officers).

7. Ericsson, Krampe, and Tesch-Römer 1993.

8. *Id.*

9. Wamsley and Stickgold 2011.

10. Killgore et al 2007.

11. Killgore et al 2008. *See also* Wilckens et al 2014 (sleep loss impairs working memory and verbal fluency).

12. "Dexies" is a nickname for dextroamphetamine, also known as Dexedrine. Modafinil is a stimulant.

13. Killgore, Grugle, and Balkin 2012.

14. Ferrara et al 2015 (emphasis in original).

15. Baglioni et al 2010.

16. Beattie et al 2014.

11. Who's on Top

1. *See* Barnes et al 2014 (managers more abusive when sleep deprived). *See also* Weaver 2015 (leaders in negotiations during a recent Greek fiscal crisis would have been more effective if they had had more sleep).

2. *See*, e.g., Goleman 2005.

3. Fleischman 2004:63 (Gage lost the ability to be an effective foreman).

4. *See*, e.g., Morrell and Capparell 2002:41.

5. Connolly, Ruderman, and Leslie 2014.

6. *See* O'Reilly and Dugard 2014:33 (Patton would read when he experienced difficulty sleeping).

7. Sundelin et al 2013 (sleep deprivation degrades features of the face and impedes communication).

8. *See* Dinges et al 1997 (adequate sleep reduces mood disturbances).

9. O'Reilly and Dugard 2014:33.

10. Aristotle 1877:224 (importance of avoiding emotions that distort good judgment).

11. *See* Miller, Shattuck, and Matsangas 2011 (82.6 percent of Army officers sleep deprived). "You have no idea how many Republican and Democratic members of the House and Senate are chronically sleep deprived," says Bill Clinton. "I know this is an unusual theory, but I do believe sleep deprivation has a lot to do with some of the edginess of Washington today" (Leibovich 2008).

12. Giam 1997. *See also* Boonstra et al 2007 (sleep deprivation increases adenosine levels, causing reduced cortical responsiveness to incoming stimuli and reduced attention).

13. Luxton et al 2011 (2,738 soldiers surveyed; 72 percent slept less than six hours a night).

14. *See* Vorobyev et al 2015 (risky decision making associated with high thalamic activation).

15. *See* Liu et al 2014 (sleep deprivation reduces thalamic gray matter).

16. *See* Ritter and Dijksterhuis 2014 (unconscious processes contribute to creative thinking).

17. Alger et al 2015. *See also* Payne and Kensinger 2010 (sleep reorders memory so you selectively remember important details and forget the unimportant).

18. Choi 2010.

19. Connolly, Ruderman, and Leslie 2014.

12. Get a Room

1. *See* Vohs, Redden, and Rahinel 2013 (disorderliness associated with creativity).

2. But *see* Vohs, Redden, and Rahinel 2013 (people in disorderly rooms are more creative).

3. These recommendations may prove especially important if predictions of an imminent ice age materialize (*see* Casey 2014).

4. *See* Brunborg et al 2011 (computers and mobile phones disturb sleep).

5. Wilkinson and Campbell 1984 (lowering bedroom noise by 5.8 decibels increases stage 4 NREM sleep).

13. Sleep Envy

1. The International Classification of Sleep Disorders, American Sleep Disorders Association 1990:28.

2. Jacobs 2004.

3. The American Board of Sleep Medicine keeps a list of certified sleep specialists who provide CBT services. From an investment perspective, in the long run CBT-I is less expensive than continued use of prescription sleeping medications, not to mention the costs of personal and professional problems that often accompany insomnia.

14. Good in Bed

1. *Macbeth*. II.ii.

2. Sleep apnea, a condition in which people stop breathing during periods of deep sleep, is often associated with obesity and may considerably threaten the ability to work even years before diagnosis. Men and women with sleep apnea lost 1.6 to 1.8 times more workdays, respectively, during the five years prior to diagnosis than their counterparts without sleep apnea, according to an assessment of work absences among public sector employees in Finland (Palamaner Subash Shantha et al 2015).

3. *See* Sampol et al 2010 (alcohol increases risk of death from apnea).

4. Quan et al 2014.

5. Krishnan et al 2014.

6. Luboshitzky et al 2002 (apnea may contribute to low testosterone).

7. *See*, e.g., Uyrum et al 2015 (genetic basis of apnea).

8. This is the treatment that Red Sox first baseman Mike Napoli had, which was very successful for him.

9. Another machine, which doesn't use a mask but a soft mouthpiece and oral pressure therapy instead, has also been found to be effective for mild to severe apnea (Colrain et al 2013).

10. Mansukhani, Wang, and Somers 2015.

11. If ferritin levels are low normal, the addition of iron may help relieve the discomfort. Treatment generally requires the use of medications such as dopamine agonists (ropinirole and pramipexole), benzodiazepines (e.g., clonazepam) or opioids (e.g., Codeine). The discomfort can be initiated or worsened with certain medications including the SSRI antidepressants and antihistamines.

12. Parish 2013.

13. The Epworth Sleepiness Scale is a tool used by sleep specialists to assess daytime sleepiness.

15. Sleep, Drugs, and Rock & Roll

1. You can take a direct-to-consumer genetic test from 23andMe to find out if you're a rapid or a slow caffeine metabolizer. *See also* Cornelis et al 2006 (rapid metabolizers of caffeine reduce heart attack risk by consuming the drug).

2. Killgore, Grugle, and Balkin 2012.

3. Kripke, Langer, and Kline 2012.

16. Sleeping with the Enemy

1. Selye 1978 (emphasis in original).

2. Selye 1978:63.

3. Sapolsky 2004:233 (CIF turns off glucocorticoid secretion).

4. For the purposes of illustration, we talked about stepping on the mice's feet, but actually the scientists applied an electric shock. Same effect: the mice were highly stressed (*see* Tache, Morley, and Brown 2012, and *see* Redei and Endroczi 1982).

17. How about a Quickie?

1. *See* Dinges et al 1997 (two full nights needed to recover for seven days of sleep restricted 33 percent below habitual sleep duration).

2. Caldwell, Caldwell, and Schmidt 2008 (strategic napping has value).

3. Faraut et al 2015.

4. *Id.*

5. Takahashi 2003. *See also* Dhand and Sohal 2006 (frequent naps and naps longer than thirty minutes lead to adverse long-term health effects).

6. Signal et al 2009.

7. Dhand and Sohal 2006 (sleep inertia occurs primarily with naps over thirty minutes).

8. Hartzler 2014 (naps good for pilots despite sleep inertia).

9. Dhand and Sohal 2006.

10. Hayashi, Motoyoshi, and Hori 2005.

11. Dhand and Sohal 2006.

12. Dinges et al 1987.

13. *Id.* (napping prior to a night of sleep loss).

14. *See* Hartzler 2014.

15. *Id. See also* Roach et al 2011 (long-haul pilots use in-flight sanctioned napping as a fatigue countermeasure). *See* www.jamesmaas.com for more about how naps, especially power naps, can help athletes and others.

16. Signal et al 2009.

17. Karhula et al 2013.

18. Takeyama, Kubo, and Itani 2005. *See also* Oriyama, Miyakoshi, and Kobayashi 2014 (two naps better than one for nightshift nurses).

19. Castillo 2011:128.

20. Waterhouse et al 2007.

21. Mednick et al 2008.

18. Sleep Habits of Highly Effective People

1. Sleep hygiene rules by themselves are often not effective, and at times can even be counterproductive, for people suffering from insomnia. This may come as a shock, especially as virtually every popular article written on insomnia is basically limited to a discussion of sleep hygiene rules. The reason for the ineffectiveness of following sleep hygiene rules for treating insomnia is that insomnia is very different from normal sleep. For example, when treating those who are having trouble with normal sleep, we talk about the importance of getting enough sleep, prioritizing sleep, meeting sleep need, etc. But with insomnia patients, we often do just the opposite. These patients feel they need more sleep than they are getting, but we are not concerned about bedtimes with them. In fact, when we recommend sleep restriction therapy to insomniacs, we actually will limit the amount of time spent in bed to much lower than sleep need. We try to take to take the focus off of sleep and instead place it clearly on the *need* for sleep. Insomnia is covered in more detail in Chapter 13.

Insomnia patients are different, and we have attempted to note throughout this chapter where advice that would be good for normal sleepers is actually counter to what we recommend for insomnia. We include this chapter on sleep hygiene because these rules are an important starting point in getting your sleep back. However, it appears that sleep hygiene alone is neither sufficient nor necessary for good sleep to occur for those with insomnia.

2. Steven Cherniske's *Caffeine Blues* (1998) is a good overview of the dangers of caffeine. A contrasting perspective is Bennett Allen Weinberg and Bonnie Bealer's *The Caffeine Advantage* (2002).

3. *See,* e.g., Wiley and Formby 2001, who mount a devastating critique of the insidious way that lightbulbs, computers, and television screens disrupt our natural sleep cycle and wreak havoc with our health.

4. If you have this type of insomnia, you may notice that you get drowsy or even fall asleep on the couch, but once you get up and go to bed, you can't sleep. People with this problem sleep better in hotels (at least the first night). They also sleep well during sleep studies, much to their embarrassment. Part of the reason for this is that hotels and sleep labs don't have the same negative stimulus value as their home bedroom. Unfamiliar environments invoke different (usually positive) expectations about sleep and as a result, it happens.

5. Tagaya, Murayama, and Fukase 2015.

6. Falbe et al 2015.

7. An exception was research by Gitanjali, in which no evidence was found for the positive effect of music on sleep (1998).

8. *See* www.007museum.com/Kennedy_Obama.htm. *See also* Dallek 2003:362. On Kennedy's insomnia, see O'Brien 2005:228, 759, and Kennedy 1956:65.

9. Foster et al 1991.

10. Czeisler et al 1995, and Klerman et al 2002.

11. Provencio et al 1998.

12. Brown and Robinson 2004. Sunlight is also replete with these stimulating blue wavelengths, which is why we can say with confidence that humans have evolved to be awake during the time the sun is in the sky. These facts can also be used to demonstrate that humans are nocturnal sleepers, and that shift work is an unnatural state for us.

13. Harvard Health Letter 2012.

14. Counting sheep works by involving both brain hemispheres, which can sometimes prevent the kind of mentation that produces insomnia.

BIBLIOGRAPHY

Abbasi, B., M. Kimiagar, K. Sadeghniiat, M. M. Shirazi, M. Hedayati, and
B. Rashidkhani
2012. "The effect of magnesium supplementation on primary insomnia in
elderly: a double-blind placebo-controlled clinical trial." J Res Med Sci. Dec;
17(12):1161–9.

Akerstedt, T., A. Knutsson, P. Westerholm, T. Theorell, L. Alfredsson, and G. Kecklund
2002. "Sleep disturbances, work stress and work hours: a cross-sectional study."
J Psychosom Res. Sep; 53(3):741–8.

Akerstedt, T., B. Arnetz, G. Ficca, L. E. Paulsson, and A. Kallner
1999. "A 50-Hz electromagnetic field impairs sleep." J Sleep Res. Mar; 8(1):
77–81.

Alger, S. E., A. M. Chambers, T. Cunningham, and J. D. Payne
2015. "The role of sleep in human declarative memory consolidation." Curr Top
Behav Neurosci. 25:269–306.

Altman, Lawrence
1992. "Bush is to avoid using controversial sleeping pill." *New York Times*. Feb 6.

Alvarez, G. G., and N. T. Ayas
2004. "The impact of daily sleep duration on health: a review of the literature."
Prog Cardiovasc Nurs. Spring; 19(2):56–9.

Ancoli-Israel, S., K. E. Vanover, D. M. Weiner, R. E. Davis, and D. P. van Kammen
2011. "Pimavanserin tartrate, a 5-HT(2A) receptor inverse agonist, increases
slow wave sleep as measured by polysomnography in healthy adult volunteers."
Sleep Med. Feb; 12(2):134–41.

Antony, J. W., E. W. Gobel, J. K. O'Hare, P. J. Reber, and K. A. Paller
2012. "Cued memory reactivation during sleep influences skill learning." Nature
Neuroscience. 15:1114–6.

Aristotle
1877. *Aristotle's Politics*. W. E. Bolland, trans. London: Longmans, Green and
Co.

Ascher-Walsh, Rebecca
2012. "Jennifer Lopez's 5 beauty tips." WebMD. Feb 1.

Axelsson, John, et al
2010. "Beauty Sleep: experimental Study on the Perceived Health and
Attractiveness of Sleep Deprived People." BMJ. 341:c6614.

Baglioni, C., K. Spiegelhalder, C. Lombardo, and D. Riemann
2010. "Sleep and emotions: a focus on insomnia." Sleep Med Rev. Aug;
14(4):227–38.

Barnes, C. M., B. C. Gunia, and D. T. Wagner
    2015. "Sleep and moral awareness." J Sleep Res. Apr; 24(2):181–8.
Barnes, Christopher, Lucianetti Lorenzo, Bhave Devasheesh, and Michael Christian
    2014. "You wouldn't like me when I'm sleepy: leader sleep, daily abusive super-
    vision, and work unit engagement." Academy of Management Journal, Nov 3.
    amj.2013.1063.
Barrett, Deirdre
    2001. *The Committee of Sleep: How Artists, Scientists, and Athletes Use Dreams for
    Creative Problem-Solving—and How You Can Too*. New York: Crown.
Bartell, S., and S. Zallek
    2006. "Intravenous magnesium sulfate may relieve restless legs syndrome in
    pregnancy."
    J Clin Sleep Med. Apr 15; 2(2):187–8.
Bartram, Cotruvo J. (ed)
    2009. "Calcium and magnesium in drinking water: public health significance."
    Geneva, Switzerland: World Health Organization.
Bastuji, H., and M. Jouvet
    1985. [Value of the sleep diary in the study of vigilance dis]. [Article in French]
    Electroencephalogr Clin Neurophysiol. Apr; 60(4):299–305.
Batéjat, D. M., and D. O. Lagarde
    1999. "Naps and modafinil as countermeasures for the effects of sleep depriva-
    tion on cognitive performance." Aviat Space Environ Med. May; 70(5):493–8.
Bauerlein, Mark
    2008. *The Dumbest Generation: How the Digital Age Stupefies Young Americans
    and Jeopardizes Our Future (Or, Don't Trust Anyone Under 30)*. New York:
    Tarcher/Penguin.
Baumann, M., S. Peck, C. Collins, and G. Eades
    2013. "The meaning and value of taking part in a person-centred arts
    programme to hospital-based stroke patients: findings from a qualitative study."
    Disabil Rehabil. Feb; 35(3):244–56.
BBC News
    2005. "Many politicians sleep deprived." Mar 1.
Beattie, L., S. D. Kyle, C. A. Espie, and S. M. Biello
    2014. "Social interactions, emotion and sleep: a systematic review and research
    agenda." Sleep Med Rev. Dec 27; 24C:83–100.
Belenky, G., et al
    2003. "Patterns of performance degradation and restoration during sleep
    restriction and subsequent recovery: a sleep dose-response study." J Sleep Res.
    Mar; 12(1):1–12.
Benson, Herbert
    1975. *The Relaxation Response*. New York: Morrow.

Benton, M. L., and N. S. Friedman
    2013. "Treatment of obstructive sleep apnea syndrome with nasal positive
    airway pressure improves golf performance." J Clin Sleep Med. Dec 15;
    9(12):1237–42.
Better Sleep Council, The
    2014. "Starving for sleep: America's Hunger Games."
Blum, K., et al
    1993. "Genetic predisposition in alcoholism: association of the D2 dopamine
    receptor TaqI B1 RFLP with severe alcoholics." Alcohol. Jan–Feb;10(1):59–67.
Boonstra, T. W., J. F. Stins, A. Daffertshofer, and P. J. Beek
    2007. "Effects of sleep deprivation on neural functioning: an integrative review."
    Cell Mol Life Sci. Apr; 64(7–8):934–46.
Boubekri, Mohamed, et al
    2014. "Impact of windows and daylight exposure on overall health and sleep
    quality of office workers: a case-control pilot study." J Clin Sleep Med. Jun 15;
    10(6):603–11.
Brainard, G. C., B. A. Richardson, T. S. King, and R. J. Reiter
    1984. "The influence of different light spectra on the suppression of pineal
    melatonin content in the Syrian hamster." Brain Res. Mar 5; 294(2):333–9.
Braun, Lesley, and Marc Cohen
    2015. *Herbs and Natural Supplements, Vol. 2: An Evidence-Based Guide*. 4th ed.
    New York: Churchill Livingstone.
Bremner, W. J.
    2010. "Testosterone deficiency and replacement in older men." N Engl J Med.
    Jul 8; 363(2):189–91.
Brown, R. Lane, and Phyllis R. Robinson
    2004. "Melanopsin—shedding light on the elusive circadian photopigment."
    Chronobiol Int. Mar; 21(2):189–204. PMC.
Brunborg, G. S., et al
    2011. "The relationship between media use in the bedroom, sleep habits and
    symptoms of insomnia." J Sleep Res. Dec; 20(4):569–75.
Bureau of Labor Statistics
    2015. "Labor force statistics from the current population survey." US Dept. of
    Labor.
Burgess, Anthony
    2012. *A Clockwork Orange*. Restored text ed. New York: Norton.
Burke, T. M., F. A. Scheer, J. M. Ronda, C. A. Czeisler, and K. P. Wright Jr.
    2015. "Sleep inertia, sleep homeostatic and circadian influences on higher-order
    cognitive functions." J Sleep Res. Aug; 24(4):364–71.
Burkhart, K., and J. R. Phelps
    2009. "Amber lenses to block blue light and improve sleep: a randomized trial."
    Chronobiol Int. Dec; 26(8):1602–12.

Burnette, Cheryl
    2011. "Sleep education and other support significantly reduces turnover among
    first-year nurses." US Dept. of Health & Human Services, Agency for
    Healthcare Research and Quality.
Bush, George H. W.
    2013. *All the Best: My Life in Letters and Other Writings*, rev. ed. New York:
    Scribner.

Cai, J. D., S. A. Mednick, E. M. Harrison, J. C. Kanady, and S. C. Mednick
    2009. "REM, not incubation, improves creativity by priming associate
    networks." Proc Natl Acad Sci U S A, 106:10130–4.
Cajochen, C., et al
    2013. "Evidence that the lunar cycle influences human sleep." Curr Biol. Aug 5;
    23(15):1485–8.
Caldwell, J. A., J. L. Caldwell, and R. M. Schmidt
    2008. "Alertness management strategies for operational contexts." Sleep Med
    Rev. Aug; 12(4):257–73.
Campbell, S. S., M. D. Stanchina, J. R. Schlang, and P. J. Murphy
    2011. "Effects of a month long napping regimen in older individuals."
    J Am Geriatr Soc. Feb; 59(2):224–32.
Carrère, Emmanuel
    2005. *I Am Alive and You Are Dead: A Journey into the Mind of Philip K. Dick.*
    Timothy Bent, trans. New York: Picador.
Carskadon, Mary A., E. J. Orav, and W. C. Dement
    1983. "Evolution of sleep and daytime sleepiness in adolescents." In *Sleep/Wake
    Disorders: Natural History, Epidemiology, and Long-Term Evolution.*
    C. Guilleminault and E. Lugaresi, eds. New York: Raven Press. 201–16.
Casey, John
    2014. *Dark Winter: How the Sun is Causing a 30-Year Cold Spell.* Boca Raton:
    Humanix Books.
Castillo, Luis
    2011. *Clubhouse Confidential: A Yankee Bat Boy's Insider Tale of Wild Nights,
    Gambling, and Good Times with Modern Baseball's Greatest Team.* With William
    Cane. New York: St. Martin's.
Chang, A. M., D. Aeschbach, J. F. Duffy, and C. A. Czeisler
    2015. "Evening use of light-emitting eReaders negatively affects sleep,
    circadian timing, and next-morning alertness." Proc Natl Acad Sci U S A.
    Jan 27; 112(4):1232–7.
Cherniske, Stephen
    1998. *Caffeine Blues: Wake Up to the Hidden Dangers of America's #1 Drug.* New
    York: Warner Books.

Chervin, R. D., D. L. Ruzicka, A. Vahabzadeh, M. C. Burns, J. W. Burns, and
S. R. Buchman
2013. "The face of sleepiness: improvement in appearance after treatment of
sleep apnea." J Clin Sleep Med. Sep; 9(9):845–52.

Choi, Charles
2010. "Sleep cherry-picks memories, boosts cleverness." National Geographic
News. Dec 2.

Cohen, D. A., W. Wang, J. K. Wyatt, R. E. Kronauer, D. J. Dijk, C. A. Czeisler, and E.
B. Klerman
2010. "Uncovering residual effects of chronic sleep loss on human performance."
Sci Transl Med. Jan 13; 2(14).

Colrain, Ian M., et al
2013. "A multicenter evaluation of oral pressure therapy for the treatment of
obstructive sleep apnea." Sleep Med. Sep; 14(9):830–7.

Colten, H. R., and B. M. Altevogt (eds)
2006. "Extent and Health Consequences of Chronic Sleep Loss and Sleep
Disorders." In *Sleep Disorders and Sleep Deprivation: An Unmet Public Health
Problem.* Washington, DC: National Academies Press.

Connolly, Carol, Marian Ruderman, and Jean Brittain Leslie
2014. "Sleep well, lead well: how better sleep can improve leadership, boost
productivity, and spark innovation." Center for Creative Leadership.

Coren, Stanley
1999. "Sleepiness cycles: the hidden danger." Address at the Canadian Aviation
Safety Seminar, Vancouver, British Columbia. May.

Cornelis, M. C., A. El-Sohemy, E. K. Kabagambe, and H. Campos
2006. "Coffee, CYP1A2 genotype, and risk of myocardial infarction." JAMA.
Mar 8; 295(10):1135–41.

Correia, H. R., S. C. Balseiro, and M. L. de Areia
2005. "Are genes of human intelligence related to the metabolism of thyroid
and steroids hormones?—endocrine changes may explain human evolution and
higher intelligence." Med Hypotheses; 65(6):1016–23.

Crowther, D., T. Wilkinson, P. Biddulph, T. Oreszczyn, S. Pretlove, and I. Ridley
2006. "A simple model for predicting the effect of hygrothermal conditions on
populations of house dust mite *Dermatophagoides pteronyssinus* (Acari: Pyro-
glyphidae)." Exp Appl Acarol. 39(2):127–48.

Czeisler, Charles A., et al
1995. "Suppression of melatonin secretion in some blind patients by exposure to
bright light." N Engl J Med. Jan 5; 332(1):6–11.

Dallek, Robert
2003. *An Unfinished Life: John F. Kennedy, 1917–1963.* New York: Little, Brown.

Dauvilliers, Y., and M. Tafti
    2008. "The genetic basis of sleep disorders." Curr Pharm Des. 14(32):3386–95.
Dean, Carolyn
    2006. *The Magnesium Miracle*, rev. ed. New York: Ballantine.
de la Iglesia, H. O., E. Fernández-Duque, D. A. Golombek, N. Lanza, J. F. Duffy, C.
    A. Czeisler, and C. R. Valeggia 2015. "Access to electric light is associated with
    shorter sleep duration in a traditionally hunter-gatherer community."
    J Biol Rhythms. Jun 18.
Dement, William
    1999. *The Promise of Sleep*. New York: Delacorte.
Dhand, R., and H. Sohal
    2006. "Good sleep, bad sleep! The role of daytime naps in healthy adults."
    Curr Opin Pulm Med. Nov; 12(6):379–82.
Dick, Philip K.
    2011. *The Three Stigmata of Palmer Eldritch*. New York: Mariner Books.
Dinges, D. F., et al
    1997. "Cumulative sleepiness, mood disturbance, and psychomotor vigilance
    performance decrements during a week of sleep restricted to 4–5 hours per
    night." Sleep. Apr; 20(4):267–77.
Dinges, D. F., M. T. Orne, W. G. Whitehouse, and E. C. Orne
    1987. "Temporal placement of a nap for alertness: contributions of circadian
    phase and prior wakefulness." Sleep. Aug; 10(4):313–29.
Duhigg, Charles
    2014. *The Power of Habit*. New York: Random House.

Eickhoff, E., K. Yung, D. L. Davis, F. Bishop, W. P. Klam, and A. P. Doan
    2015. "Excessive video game use, sleep deprivation, and poor work performance
    among US Marines treated in a military mental health clinic: a case series."
    Mil Med. Jul; 180(7):e839–43.
Elliot, Danielle
    2014. "The doctor who coaches athletes on sleep." *Atlantic*. Apr 23.
Ericsson, K. Anders, Ralf T. Krampe, and Clemens Tesch-Römer
    1993. "The role of deliberate practice in the acquisition of expert performance."
    Psychol Rev. 100(3):363–406.
Eriksson, M., U. Berggren, K. Blennow, C. Fahlke, J. E. Månsson, and J. Balldin
    2000. "Alcoholics with the dopamine receptor DRD2 A1 allele have lower
    platelet monoamine oxidase-B activity than those with the A2 allele: a
    preliminary study." Alcohol Alcohol. Sep–Oct; 35(5):493–8.
Erlacher, Daniel
    2012. "Practicing in dreams can improve your performance." Harv Bus Rev.
    Apr; 90(4):30–1.

Falbe, J., et al
    2015. "Sleep duration, restfulness, and screens in the sleep environment."
    Pediatrics. Feb; 135(2):e367–75.

Faraut, B., et al
    2015. "Napping reverses the salivary interleukin-6 and urinary
    norepinephrine changes induced by sleep restriction." J Clin Endocrinol Metab.
    Mar; 100(3):e416–26.

Ferber, Richard
    2006. *Solve Your Child's Sleep Problems: New, Revised, and Expanded Edition.*
    New York: Touchstone.

Ferini-Strambi, L., M. L. Fantini, and C. Castronovo
    2004. "Epidemiology of obstructive sleep apnea syndrome." Minerva Med. Jun;
    95(3):187–202.

Ferrara, Michele, et al
    2015. "Gender differences in sleep deprivation effects on risk and
    inequality aversion: evidence from an economic experiment." PLoS ONE.
    Mar 20; 10(3):e0120029.

Fleischman, John
    2004. *Phineas Gage: A Gruesome but True Story about Brain Science.* Boston:
    Houghton Mifflin Harcourt.

Ford, Earl S., and Ali H. Mokdad
    2003. "Dietary magnesium intake in a national sample of US adults."
    J Nutr. 133(9):2879–82.

Foster, R. G., et al
    1991. "Circadian photoreception in the retinally degenerate mouse (rd/rd)."
    J Comp Physiol A. Jul; 169(1):39–50.

Friman, P. C., et al
    1999. "The bedtime pass: an approach to bedtime crying and leaving the room."
    Arch Pediatr Adolesc Med. Oct; 153(10):1027–9.

Fullagar, H. H., R. Duffield, S. Skorski, A. J. Coutts, R. Julian, T. Meyer
    2015. "Sleep and recovery in team sport: current sleep-related issues facing
    professional team-sport athletes." Int J Sports Physiol Perform.
    Nov; 10(8):950-7.

Gartner, John D.
    2011. *The Hypomanic Edge: The Link Between (a Little) Craziness and (a Lot of)*
    Success in America. New York: Simon & Schuster.

George, Nancy M., and Jean E. Davis.
    2013. "Assessing sleep in adolescents through a better understanding of sleep
    physiology." Am J Nurs. 113(6):26–31.

Giam, G. C.
    1997. "Effects of sleep deprivation with reference to military operations."
    Ann Acad Med, Singapore. Jan; 26(1):88–93.

Gibson, A. A., et al
    2015. "Do ketogenic diets really suppress appetite? A systematic review and meta-analysis." Obes Rev. Jan; 16(1):64–76.
Gitanjali, B.
    1998. "Effect of the Karnatic music raga 'Neelambari' on sleep architecture." Indian J Physiol Pharmacol. Jan; 42(1):119–22.
Goleman, Daniel
    2005. *Emotional Intelligence*. New York: Bantam.
Gross, Lee, et al
    2004. "Increased consumption of refined carbohydrates and the epidemic of type 2 diabetes in the United States: an ecologic assessment." Am J Clin Nutr. 79(5):774–9.
Guilleminault, C.
    1990. "Benzodiazepines, breathing, and sleep." Am J Med. Mar 2; 88(3A):25S–28S.

Hale-Evans, Ron
    2006. *Mind Performance Hacks: Tips & Tools for Overclocking Your Brain*. Sebastopol, CA: O'Reilly Media.
Hall, Alena
    2015. "14 highly successful people who prioritize a good night's sleep." Huffington Post. Jul 27.
Hartzler, B. M.
    2014. "Fatigue on the flight deck: the consequences of sleep loss and the benefits of napping." Accid Anal Prev. Jan; 62:309–18.
Harvard Health Letter
    2012. "Blue light has a dark side." May 1.
Harvard Health Publications
    2007. "Repaying your sleep debt." Aug 1.
Hasler, B. P., and W. M. Troxel
    2010. "Couples' nighttime sleep efficiency and concordance: evidence for bidirectional associations with daytime relationship functioning." Psychosom Med. Oct; 72(8):794–801.
Hatfield, Heather
    2007. "How to sleep like an Olympic athlete." WebMD. Jan 1.
Hayashi, M., A. Masuda, and T. Hori
    2003. "The alerting effects of caffeine, bright light and face washing after a short daytime nap." Clin Neurophysiol. Dec; 114(12):2268–78.
Hayashi, M., M. Watanabe, and T. Hori
    1999. "The effects of a 20 min nap in the mid-afternoon on mood, performance and EEG activity." Clin Neurophysiol. Feb; 110(2):272–9.

Hayashi, M., N. Motoyoshi, and T. Hori
      2005. "Recuperative power of a short daytime nap with or without stage 2
      sleep." Sleep. Jul; 28(7):829–36.

Holland, Julie (ed)
      2010. *The Pot Book: A Complete Guide to Cannabis, Its Role in Medicine, Politics,*
      Science, and Culture. Rochester, VT: Park Street Press.

Horne, J. A.
      2015. "Human REM sleep: influence on feeding behaviour, with clinical
      implications." Sleep Med. Aug; 16(8):910–6.

Hornyak, M., U. Voderholzer, F. Hohagen, M. Berger, and D. Riemann
      1998. "Magnesium therapy for periodic leg movements-related insomnia and
      restless legs syndrome: an open pilot study." Sleep. Aug 1; 21(5):501–5.

Howard, Hilary
      2014. "She wasn't called 'Sleepless Beauty': want a good night's sleep? make a
      plan." *New York Times.* Jun 19.

Huang, H. W., et al
      2015. "Effect of oral melatonin and wearing earplugs and eye masks on
      nocturnal sleep in healthy subjects in a simulated intensive care unit
      environment: which might be a more promising strategy for ICU sleep
      deprivation?" Crit Care. Mar 19; 19(1):124.

Hubpages
      2014. "Ten things you didn't know about Babe Ruth." Aug 17.

Huffington, Arianna
      2015. "My Q and A with sleep expert Mathias Basner on the science of sleep."
      Huffpost Healthy Living. Jul 8.

Huntford, Roland
      1984. *Shackleton.* New York: Carroll & Graf.

Hyman, Mark
      2012. *The Blood Sugar Solution: The UltraHealthy Program for Losing Weight,*
      Preventing Disease, and Feeling Great Now! New York: Little, Brown.

Jackson, Joe
      2007. *A World on Fire: A Heretic, an Aristocrat, and the Race to Discover Oxygen.*
      New York: Penguin.

Jacobs, G. D., E. F. Pace-Schott, R. Stickgold, and M. W. Otto
      2004. "Cognitive behavior therapy and pharmacotherapy for insomnia: a
      randomized controlled trial and direct comparison." Arch Intern Med. Sep 27;
      164(17):1888–96.

Jespersen, K. V., J. Koenig, P. Jennum, and P. Vuust
      2015. "Music for insomnia in adults." Cochrane Database Syst Rev. Aug 13;
      8:CD010459.

Jones, Christopher R., Angela L. Huang, Louis J. Ptáček, and Ying-Hui Fu
    2013. "Genetic basis of human circadian rhythm disorders." Exp Neurol. Jul;
    243:28–33.
Jones, Jeffrey
    2013. "In US, 40% Get Less Than Recommended Amount of Sleep." Gallup
    poll.
Jones, Maggie
    2011. "How little sleep can you get away with?" *New York Times*. Apr 15.
Juliff, L. E., S. L. Halson, and J. J. Peiffer
    2015. "Understanding sleep disturbance in athletes prior to important
    competitions." J Sci Med Sport. Jan; 18(1):13–8.

Kalmbach, D. A., J. T. Arnedt, V. Pillai, and J. A. Ciesla
    2015. "The impact of sleep on female sexual response and behavior: a pilot
    study." J Sex Med. May; 12(5):1221–32.
Kalmbach, D. A., V. Pillai, T. Roth, and C. L. Drake
    2014. "The interplay between daily affect and sleep: a 2-week study of young
    women." J Sleep Res. Dec; 23(6):636–45.
Kamdar, B. B., K. A. Kaplan, E. J. Kezirian, W. C. Dement
    2004. "The impact of extended sleep on daytime alertness, vigilance, and mood."
    Sleep Med. Sep; 5(5):441–8.
Karhula, K., et al
    2013. "Job strain, sleep and alertness in shift working health care
    professionals—a field study." Ind Health. 51(4):406–16.
Katz, A. S., N. P. Pronk, and M. Lowry
    2014. "The association between optimal lifestyle-related health behaviors and
    employee productivity." J Occup Environ Med. Jul; 56(7):708–13.
Kennedy, John F.
    1956. *Profiles in Courage*. New York: Harper & Brothers.
Killgore, W. D.
    2010. "Effects of sleep deprivation on cognition." Prog Brain Res. 185:105–29.
Killgore, W. D., D. B. Killgore, L. M. Day, C. Li, G. H. Kamimori, and T. J. Balkin
    2007. "The effects of 53 hours of sleep deprivation on moral judgment." Sleep.
    Mar; 30(3):345–52.
Killgore, W. D., E. T. Kahn-Greene, E. L. Lipizzi, R. A. Newman, G. H. Kamimori,
    and T. J. Balkin
    2008. "Sleep deprivation reduces perceived emotional intelligence and
    constructive thinking skills." Sleep Med. Jul; 9(5):517–26.
Killgore, W. D., N. L. Grugle, and T. J. Balkin
    2012. "Gambling when sleep deprived: don't bet on stimulants." Chronobiol Int.
    Feb; 29(1):43–54.

King, D. E., A. G. Mainous III, M. E. Geesey, and R. F. Woolson
    2005. "Dietary magnesium and C-reactive protein levels." J Am Coll Nutr. Jun;
    24(3):166–71.
Kling, R.N., C.B. McLeod, and M. Koehoorn
    2010. "Sleep problems and workplace injuries in Canada." Sleep. May 1; 33(5):
    611–8.
Kivimäki, Mika, et al
    2011. "Using additional information on working hours to predict coronary heart
    disease: a cohort study." Ann Intern Med. 154(7):457–63. PMC.
Klerman, E. B., et al
    2002. "Photic resetting of the human circadian pacemaker in the absence of
    conscious vision." J Biol Rhythms. Dec; 17(6):548–55.
Knutson, Kristen L., et al
    2010. "Trends in the prevalence of short sleepers in the USA: 1975–2006."
    Sleep. 33(1): 37–45.
Kripke, D. F., R. D. Langer, and L. E. Kline
    2012. "Hypnotics' association with mortality or cancer: a matched cohort study."
    BMJ Open. Feb 27; 2(1):e000850.
Krishnan, V., S. Dixon-Williams, and J. D. Thornton
    2014. "Where there is smoke . . . there is sleep apnea: exploring the relationship
    between smoking and sleep apnea." Chest. Dec; 146(6):1673–80.
Kroese, F. M., C. Evers, M. A. Adriaanse, D. T. de Ridder
    2014. "Bedtime procrastination: a self-regulation perspective on sleep
    insufficiency in the general population." J Health Psychol. Jul 4.
Kucharczyk, E. R., K. Morgan, and A. P. Hall
    2012. "The occupational impact of sleep quality and insomnia symptoms."
    Sleep Med Rev. Dec; 16(6):547–59.
Kushida, Clete A. (ed)
    2004. "Sleep Deprivation: Clinical Issues, Pharmacology, and Sleep Loss
    Effects." In *Lung Biology in Health and Disease.* Vol. 193. Boca Raton, FL: CRC
    Press.
Kyle, S. D., L. Beattie, K. Spiegelhalder, Z. Rogers, and C. A. Espie
    2014. "Altered emotion perception in insomnia disorder." Sleep. Apr 1;
    37(4):775–83.

LaBerge, Stephen
    1985. *Lucid Dreaming.* Los Angeles: J. P. Tarcher.
Lallukka, Tea, et al
    2014. "Sleep and sickness absence: a nationally representative register-based
    follow-up study." Sleep. Sep 1; 37(9):1413–25.

Lane, M. R.
        2005. "Creativity and spirituality in nursing: implementing art in healing."
        Holist Nurs Pract. May–Jun; 19(3):122–5.
Lee, H., et al
        2015. "The effect of body posture on brain glymphatic transport." J Neurosci.
        Aug 5; 35(31):11034–44.
Leibovich, Mark
        2008. "Fatigue factor gives equal time to candidates." *New York Times.* Jan 3.
Leproult, Rachel, and Eve Van Cauter
        2011. "Effect of 1 week of sleep restriction on testosterone levels in young
        healthy men" JAMA. Jun 1; 305(21): 2173–4.
Levendowski, D. J., T. Morgan, J. Montague, V. Melzer, C. Berka, and P. R. Westbrook
        2008. "Prevalence of probable obstructive sleep apnea risk and severity in a
        population of dental patients." Sleep Breath. Nov; 12(4):303–9.
Littner, M., et al
        2001. "Practice parameters for the treatment of narcolepsy: an update for 2000."
        Sleep. Jun 15; 24(4):451–66.
Liu, C., X. Z. Kong, X. Liu, R. Zhou, and B. Wu
        2014. "Long-term total sleep deprivation reduces thalamic gray matter volume
        in healthy men." Neuroreport. Mar 26; 25(5):320–3.
Lovato, N., and L. Lack
        2010. "The effects of napping on cognitive functioning." Prog Brain Res.
        185:155–66.
Luboshitzky, R., et al
        2002. "Decreased pituitary-gonadal secretion in men with obstructive sleep
        apnea." J Clin Endocrinol Metab. Jul; 87(7):3394–8.
Lucassen, Eliane A., et al
        2014. "Sleep extension improves neurocognitive functions in chronically
        sleep-deprived obese individuals." Ed. Hemachandra Reddy. PLoS ONE. Jan
        15; 9(1):e84832.
Luckhaupt, Sara E.
        2012. "Short sleep duration among workers—United States, 201." Centers for
        Disease Control and Prevention. Apr 27; 61(16):281–5.
Luxton, D. D., D. Greenburg, J. Ryan, A. Niven, G. Wheeler, and V. Mysliwiec
        2011. "Prevalence and impact of short sleep duration in redeployed OIF
        soldiers." Sleep. Sep 1; 34(9):1189–95.

Ma, N., D. F. Dinges, M. Basner, and H. Rao
        2015. "How acute total sleep loss affects the attending brain: a meta-analysis of
        neuroimaging studies." Sleep. Feb 1; 38(2):233–40.

Maas, James B.
      1988. *Power Sleep: The Revolutionary Program that Prepares Your Mind for Peak
      Performance*. New York: William Morrow.
Madera, Juan M., and Michelle R. Hebl
      2012. "Discrimination against facially stigmatized applicants in interviews: an
      eye-
      tracking and face-to-face investigation." J Appl Psychol. Mar; 97(2):317–30.
Mah, C .D., K. E. Mah, E. J. Kezirian, and W. C. Dement
      2011. "The effects of sleep extension on the athletic performance of collegiate
      basketball players." Sleep. Jul 1; 34(7):943–50.
Mander, Jerry
      1977. *Four Arguments for the Elimination of Television*. New York:
      HarperCollins.
Manfred, Tony
      2014. "Tom Brady explains why he goes to sleep at 8:30." Business Insider.
      Nov 10.
Manfredini, R., et al
      1998. "Circadian rhythms, athletic performance, and jet lag." Br. J. Sports Med.
      32(2):101–6.
Mansukhani, M. P., S. Wang, and V. K. Somers
      2015. "Sleep, death and the heart." Am J Physiol Heart Circ Physiol. Jul 17. doi:
      10.1152/ajpheart.00285.2015.
Marshall, N. S. K. K. Wong, S. R. Cullen, M. W. Knuiman, and R. R. Grunstein
      2014. "Sleep apnea and 20-year follow-up for all-cause mortality, stroke, and
      cancer incidence and mortality in the Busselton health study cohort." J Clin
      Sleep Med. Apr 15; 10(4):355–362.
McGrath, Margaux
      2015. "Unlocking the science of social jet lag and sleep: an interview with Till
      Roenneberg." Huffington Post. Jul 21.
Mednick, Sara C., et al
      2008. "Comparing the benefits of caffeine, naps and placebo on verbal, motor
      and perceptual memory." Behavioural brain research. 193(1):79–86. PMC.
Mélançon, Michel O.
      2015. "Endurance exercise, tryptophan availability to the brain, and sleep
      electro-physiology in older men." Appl Physiol Nutr Metab. 40:306.
Mendelson, M., et al
      2015. "Sleep quality, sleep duration and physical activity in obese adolescents:
      effects of exercise training." Pediatr Obes. Mar 2.
Meskó, Norbert, Tünde Paál, and Bernadett Gábor
      2012. "The face and head hair of woman: long hairstyle as an adaptive means
      of displaying phenotipic quality." Electronic International Interdisciplinary
      Conference.

Miller, N. L., L. G. Shattuck, and P. Matsangas
    2011. "Sleep and fatigue issues in continuous operations: a survey of US Army officers." Behav Sleep Med. 9(1):53–65.
Millett, Kate
    (1970) 2000. *Sexual Politics*. New York: Doubleday. Reprint, Champaign, IL: University of Illinois Press.
Mohtashami, F., A. Thiele, E. Karreman, and J. Thiel
    2014. "Comparing technical dexterity of sleep-deprived versus intoxicated surgeons." J Soc Lapro. Oct–Dec; 18(4).
Molloy, John T.
    1996. *New Women's Dress for Success*. New York: Warner Books.
Montville, Leigh
    2007. *The Big Bam: The Life and Times of Babe Ruth*. New York: Anchor.
Morrell, Margot, and Stephanie Capparell
    2002. *Shackleton's Way: Leadership Lessons from the Great Antarctic Explorer*. New York: Penguin.
Muller, M., et al
    2005. "Endogenous sex hormone levels and cognitive function in aging men: is there an optimal level?" Neurology. Mar 8; 64(5):866–71.
Mulrine, H. M., T. L. Signal, M. J. van den Berg, and P. H. Gander
    2012. "Post-sleep inertia performance benefits of longer naps in simulated nightwork and extended operations." Chronobiol Int. Nov; 29(9):1249–57.

Naiman, Rubin
    2014. *Hush: A Book of Bedtime Contemplations*. Tucson, AZ: New Moon Media.
Nielsen, T. A., D. Kuiken, G. Alain, P. Stenstrom, and R. A. Powell
    2004. "Immediate and delayed incorporations of events into dreams: further replication and implications for dream function." J Sleep Rese, 13:327–36.
Nietzsche, Friedrich
    1968. *Twilight of the Idols and the Anti-Christ*. R. J. Hollingdale, trans. Baltimore: Penguin.
Nygaard, I. H., A. Valbø, S. V. Pethick, and T. Bøhmer
    2008. "Does oral magnesium substitution relieve pregnancy-induced leg cramps?" Eur J Obstet Gynecol Reprod Biol. Nov; 141(1):23–6.

O'Brien, Michael
    2005. *John F. Kennedy: A Biography*. New York: St. Martin's.
Ødegård, Siv Steinsmo, Petter Moe Omland, Kristian Bernhard Nilsen, Marit Stjern, Gøril Bruvik Gravdahl, and Trond Sand
    2015. "The effect of sleep restriction on laser evoked potentials, thermal sensory and pain thresholds and suprathreshold pain in healthy subjects." Clin Neurophysiol. Oct; 126(10):1979-87.

Olsen, O. K., S. Pallesen, and J. Eid
    2010. "The impact of partial sleep deprivation on moral reasoning in military
    officers." Sleep. Aug; 33(8):1086–90.
Olson, Ryan, et al
    2015. "A workplace intervention improves sleep: results from the randomized
    controlled Work, Family, and Health Study." Sleep Health. 1(1):55–65.
O'Reilly, Bill, and Martin Dugard
    2014. *Killing Patton: The Strange Death of World War II's Most Audacious General.*
    New York: Henry Holt.
Oriyama, S., Y. Miyakoshi, and T. Kobayashi
    2014. "Effects of two 15-min naps on the subjective sleepiness, fatigue and
    heart rate variability of night shift nurses." Ind Health. 52(1):25–35.
Oyetakin-White, P., et al
    2015. "Does poor sleep quality affect skin aging?" Clin Exp Dermatol. Jan;
    40(1):17–22.

Palamaner Subash Shantha, G., A. A. Kumar, L. J. Cheskin, and S. B. Pancholy
    2015. "Association between sleep-disordered breathing, obstructive sleep apnea,
    and cancer incidence: a systematic review and meta-analysis." Sleep Med. Oct;
    16(10):1289–94.
Pantley, Elizabeth
    2002. *The No-Cry Sleep Solution: Gentle Ways to Help Your Baby Sleep Through the
    Night.* New York: McGraw-Hill.
Parish, James M.
    2013. "Genetic and immunologic aspects of sleep and sleep disorders." Chest.
    May; 143(5):1489–99.
Pawel, Ernst
    1984. *A Life of Franz Kafka.* New York: Farrar, Straus, and Giroux.
Payne, J. D., and E. A. Kensinger
    2010. "Sleep's role in the consolidation of emotional episodic memories." Curr
    Dir Psychol. 19(5):290–5.
Pellegrino, R., et al
    2014. "A novel BHLHE41 variant is associated with short sleep and resistance
    to sleep deprivation in humans." Sleep. Aug 1; 37(8):1327–36.
Pfann, Gerard A., Jeff E. Biddle, Daniel S. Hamermesh, and Ciska M. Bosman
    2006. "Business success and businesses' beauty capital." Economics Letters. Dec;
    93(3):201–7.
Pilcher, J. J., D. M. Morris, J. Donnelly, and H. B. Feigl
    2015. "Interactions between sleep habits and self-control." Front. Hum.
    Neurosci. May; 9:284.
Platt, Charles
    1980. *Dream Makers: The Uncommon People Who Write Science Fiction.* New York:
    Berkley Books.

Plog, Benjamin A., et al
    2015. "Biomarkers of traumatic injury are transported from brain to blood via the glymphatic system." J Neurosci. 35(2):518–526.
Poussel, M., et al
    2015. "Sleep management strategy and performance in an extreme mountain ultra-
    marathon." Res Sports Med. May; 28:1–7.
Profusek, P. J., and D. W. Rainey
    1987. "Effects of Baker-Miller pink and red on state anxiety, grip strength, and motor precision." Percept Mot Skills. Dec; 65(3):941–2.
Provencio, I., et al
    1998. "Melanopsin: an opsin in melanophores, brain, and eye." Proc Natl Acad Sci U S A. Jan 6; 95(1):340–5.
Puhan, Milo A., et al
    2006. "Didgeridoo playing as alternative treatment for obstructive sleep apnoea syndrome: randomised controlled trial." BMJ. 2006 Feb 4; 332(7536):266-70.

Quan, Z., et al
    2014. [Correlation of smoking and obstructive sleep apnea and hypopnea syndrome.] [Article in Chinese.] J of the Chinese Med Assn. Mar 18; 94(10):733–6.

Rains, V. S., T. F. Ditzler, R. D. Newsome, S. Lee-Gushi, and E. J. Morgan
    1991. "Alcohol and sleep apnea." Hawaii Med J. Aug; 50(8):282–7.
Raizen, D. M., T. B. Mason, and A. I. Pack
    2006. "Genetic basis for sleep regulation and sleep disorders." Semin Neurol. Nov; 26(5):467–83.
Rasskazova Elena, Zavalko Irina, Tkhostov Alexander, and Vladimir Dorohov
    2014. "High intention to fall asleep causes sleep fragmentation." J Sleep Res. Jun; 23(3):295–301.
Rath, Tom, and James K. Harter
    2010. Wellbeing: The Five Essential Elements. New York: Gallup Press.
Ratini, Melinda
    2014. "Human Growth Hormone (HGH)." Dec 30. WebMD.
Rechtschaffen, A.
    1971. "The Control of Sleep." In Human Behavior and Its Control, 75–92. W. A. Hunt, ed. Cambridge, MA: Shenkman.
Redei, E., and E. Endroczi
    1982. "Hypothalamic factor of inhibitory activity on pituitary adrenocortical function." In Integrative Neurohormonal Mechanism, Elsevier Science. 16:377–88.

Reich, Wilhelm
    1974. *The Sexual Revolution: Toward a Self-Regulating Character Structure.*
    New York: Farrar, Straus, and Giroux.
Rettner, Rachel
    2011. "New rules to fight crib death: breast-feeding and vaccinations."
    LiveScience.com. Oct 18.
Rhodes, G.
    2006. "The evolutionary psychology of facial beauty." Annu Rev Psychol.
    57:199–226.
Ritter, Simone M., and Ap Dijksterhuis
    2014. "Creativity—the unconscious foundations of the incubation period."
    Frontiers in Human Neuroscience. 8:215.
Roach, G. D., D. Darwent, T. L. Sletten, and D. Dawson
    2011. "Long-haul pilots use in-flight napping as a countermeasure to fatigue."
    Appl Ergon. Jan; 42(2):214–8.
Rosekind, M. R., and K. B. Gregory
    2010. "Insomnia risks and costs: health, safety, and quality of life." Am J Manag
    Care. Aug; 16(8):617–26.
Rowh, Mark
    2007. "Sleep working." Human Resources Executive Online. Feb 1.

Sallinen, M., J. Holm, K. Hirvonen, M. Härmä, J. Koskelo, M. Letonsaari,
    R. Luukkonen, J. Virkkala, and K. Müller
    2008. "Recovery of cognitive performance from sleep debt: do a short rest pause
    and a single recovery night help?" Chronobiol Int. Apr; 25(2):279–96.
Salord, N., et al
    2015. "A randomized controlled trial of continuous positive airway pressure on
    glucose tolerance in obese patients with obstructive sleep apnea." Sleep. Aug 31.
    pii: sp-00651-14.
Sampol, G., G. Rodés, J. Ríos, O. Romero, P. Lloberes, and F. Morell
    2010. [Acute hypercapnic respiratory failure in patients with sleep apneas.]
    [Article in Spanish.] Arch Bronconeumol. Sep; 46(9):466–72.
Santoso, Alex
    2007. "Proven by science: messy beds are actually healthier!" Nov 17.
Sapolsky, Robert M.
    2004. *Why Zebras Don't Get Ulcers.* 3rd ed. New York: Henry Holt and
    Company.
Sargent, C., M. Lastella, S. L. Halson, and G. D. Roach
    2014a. "The impact of training schedules on the sleep and fatigue of elite
    athletes." Chronobiol Int. Dec; 31(10):1160–8.

Sargent, C., S. Halson, and G. D. Roach
    2014b. "Sleep or swim? Early-morning training severely restricts the amount of
    sleep obtained by elite swimmers." Eur J Sport Sci. 14 Suppl 1:S310–5.

Sayón-Orea, C., M. Bes-Rastrollo, S. Carlos, J. J. Beunza, F. J. Basterra-Gortari, and
        M. A. Martínez-González
    2013. "Association between sleeping hours and siesta and the risk of obesity: the
    SUN Mediterranean Cohort." Obes Facts. 6(4):337–47.

Schlafer O., V. Wenzel, and B. Högl
    2014. [Sleep disorders among physicians on shift work.] [Article in German.]
    Anaesthesist. Nov; 63(11):844–51.

Schor, Juliet B.
    1991. *The Overworked American: The Unexpected Decline of Leisure*. New York:
    Basic Books.

Scott, Brent A., and Timothy A. Judge
    2006. "Insomnia, emotions, and job satisfaction: a multilevel study." Journal of
    Management. 32(5):622–645.

Sebo, P., B. Cerutti, and D. M. Haller
    2014. "Effect of magnesium therapy on nocturnal leg cramps: a systematic
    review of randomized controlled trials with meta-analysis using simulations."
    Fam Pract. Feb; 31(1):7–19.

Seftel, A. D., M. Kathrins, and C. Niederberger
    2015. "Critical update of the 2010 endocrine society clinical practice guidelines
    for male hypogonadism: a systematic analysis." Mayo Clin Proc. Jul 16; pii:
    S0025-6196(15)00467-X.

Selye, Hans
    1978. *The Stress of Life*. New York: McGraw-Hill.

Sergeeva, Olga A., et al
    2010. "Fragrant dioxane derivatives identify 1-subunit-containing $GABA_A$
    receptors." J Biol Chem. 285(31):23985–93. PMC.

Seystahl, Katharina, Helen Könnecke, Oguzkan Sürücü, Christian R. Baumann, and
        Rositsa Poryazova
    2014. "Development of a short sleeper phenotype after third ventriculostomy in
    a patient with ependymal cysts." J Clin Sleep Med; 10(2):211–3.

Shakespeare, William
    2003. *Macbeth*. New York: Simon & Schuster.

Sheth, B. R., D. Janvelyan, and M. Khan
    2008. "Practice makes imperfect: restorative effects of sleep on motor learning."
    PLoS One. Sep 12; 3(9):e3190.

Siegel, J. M., et al
    1998. "Monotremes and the evolution of rapid eye movement sleep." Philos
    Trans R Soc Lond B Biol Sci. Jul 29; 353(1372): 1147–57.

Signal, T. L., P. H. Gander, H. Anderson, and S. Brash
    2009. "Scheduled napping as a countermeasure to sleepiness in air traffic
    controllers." J Sleep Res. Mar; 18(1):11–19.
Sio, U. N., P. Monaghan, and T. Ormerod
    2013. "Sleep on it, but only if it is difficult: effects of sleep on problem solving."
    Mem Cognit. Feb; 41(2):159–66.
Sircus, Mark
    2011. *Transdermal Magnesium Therapy.* Bloomington, IN: iUniverse.
Sisson, Mark
    2009. *The Primal Blueprint.* Malibu, CA: Primal Nutrition, Inc.
Slama, H., G. Deliens, R. Schmitz, P. Peigneux, and R. Leproult
    2015. "Afternoon nap and bright light exposure improve cognitive flexibility
    post lunch." PLoS One. May 27; 10(5):e0125359.
Spiegel, K., E. Tasali, P. Penev, and E. Van Cauter
    2004. "Brief communication: sleep curtailment in healthy young men is associ-
    ated with decreased leptin levels, elevated ghrelin levels, and increased hunger
    and appetite." Ann Intern Med. 141:846–50.
Spiegel, K., R. Leproult, and E. Van Cauter
    1999. "Impact of sleep debt on metabolic and endocrine function." Lancet. Oct
    23; 354(9188):1435–9.
Stang, A., et al
    2007. "Daily siesta, cardiovascular risk factors, and measures of subclinical
    atherosclerosis: results of the Heinz Nixdorf Recall Study." Sleep. Sep; 30(9):
    1111–9.
Steffen, M. W., A. C. Hazelton, W. R. Moore, S. M. Jenkins, M. M. Clark, and
    P. T. Hagen
    2015. "Improving sleep: outcomes from a worksite healthy sleep program."
    J Occup Environ Med. Jan; 57(1):1–5.
St-Onge, Marie-Pierre
    2013. "The role of sleep duration in the regulation of energy balance: effects on
    energy intakes and expenditure." J Clin Sleep Med. Jan 15; 9(1):73–80.
Stumbrys, T., D. Erlacher, M. Johnson, and M. Schredl
    2014. "The phenomenology of lucid dreaming: an online survey." Am J Psychol.
    Summer; 127(2):191–204.
Sulloway, Frank
    1996. *Born to Rebel.* New York: Pantheon.
Sundelin, Tina, et al
    2013. "Cues of fatigue: effects of sleep deprivation on facial appearance." Sleep.
    36(9):1355–60.
Surani, S., V. Brito, A. Surani, and S. Ghamande
    2015. "Effect of diabetes mellitus on sleep quality." World J Diabetes. Jun 25;
    6(6):868–73.

Swerdloff, Ronald, and Christina Wang
      2011. "Testosterone treatment of older men—why are controversies created?"
      J Clin Endocrinol Metab. Sep 6; 96(1):62–5. PMC.

Tache, Yvette, John E. Morley, and Marvin R. Brown
      2012. *Neuropeptides and Stress: Proceedings of the First Hans Selye Symposium,*
      Held in Montreal in October 1986. New York: Springer.
Tagaya, H., N. Murayama, and Y. Fukase
      2015. [Circadian rhythm sleep-wake disorder (circadian rhythm sleep
      disorder).] [Article in Japanese.] Nihon Rinsho. Jun; 73(6):942–8.
Takahashi, M.
      2003. "The role of prescribed napping in sleep medicine." Sleep Med Rev. Jun;
      7(3):227–35.
Takeyama, H., T. Kubo, and T. Itani
      2005. "The nighttime nap strategies for improving night shift work in
      workplace." Ind Health. Jan; 43(1):24–9.
Tamaki, M., A. Shirota, M. Hayashi, and T. Hori
      2000. "Restorative effects of a short afternoon nap (<30 min) in the elderly on
      subjective mood, performance and EEG activity." Sleep Res Online. 3(3):131–9.
Tate, Amethyst
      2015. "Celebs aging flawlessly—halle berry, jennifer lopez, and more share their
      beauty secrets!" Ok! Magazine, Feb 10.
Thun, E., B. Bjorvatn, E. Flo, A. Harris, and S. Pallesen
      2014. "Sleep, circadian rhythms, and athletic performance." Sleep Med Rev.
      Oct; 23:1–9.
Tucker, Patty
      2013. "Preparing yourself for sleep." Sleep of Champions.

Uyrum, E., et al
      2015. "The relationship between obstructive sleep apnea syndrome and
      apolipoprotein E genetic variants." Respiration. 89(3):195–200.

Van Cauter, E., et al
      2005. "The impact of sleep deprivation on hormones and metabolism."
      Medscape Neurology. 7(1).
Van der Helm, E., N. Gujar, and M. P. Walker
      2010. "Sleep deprivation impairs the accurate recognition of human emotions."
      Sleep. Mar; 33(3):335–42.
Van Dongen, H. P., G. Maislin, J. M. Mullington, and D. F. Dinges
      2003. "The cumulative cost of additional wakefulness: dose-response effects on
      neurobehavioral functions and sleep physiology from chronic sleep restriction
      and total sleep deprivation." Sleep. Mar 15; 26(2):117–26.

Varin, C., et al
   2015. "Glucose induces slow wave sleep by exciting the sleep-promoting neurons in the ventrolateral preoptic nucleus: a new link between sleep and metabolism." J Neurosci. Jul 8; 35(27):9900–11.
Vecchio, L. M., K. P. Grace, H. Liu, S. Harding, A. D. Le, and R. L. Horner
   2009. "State-dependent vs. central motor effects of ethanol on breathing." J Appl Physiol. 108(2):387–400.
Vohs, K. D., J. P. Redden, and R. Rahinel
   2013. "Physical order produces healthy choices, generosity, and conventionality, whereas disorder produces creativity." Psychol Sci. Sep; 24(9):1860–7.
Vorobyev, V., M. S. Kwon, D. Moe, R. Parkkola, and H. Hämäläinen
   2015. "Risk-taking behavior in a computerized driving task: brain activation correlates of decision-making, outcome, and peer influence in male adolescents." PLoS One. Jun 8; 10(6):e0129516.

Wade, A. G., et al
   2010. "Nightly treatment of primary insomnia with prolonged release melatonin for 6 months: a randomized placebo controlled trial on age and endogenous melatonin as predictors of efficacy and safety." BMC Med. Aug 16; 8:51.
Wagner, U., S. Gais, H. Haider, R. Verleger, and J. Born
   2004. "Sleep inspires insight." Nature. 427:352–5.
Walker, M. P., C. Liston, J. A. Hobson, and R. Stickgold
   2002. "Cognitive flexibility across the sleep-wake cycle: REM-sleep enhancement of anagram problem solving." Cognitive Brain Res. 14:317–24.
Walker, M. P., R. Stickgold
   2005. "It's practice, with sleep, that makes perfect: implications of sleep-dependent learning and plasticity for skill performance." Clin Sports Med. Apr; 24(2):301–17.
Walker, M. P., T. Brakefield, A. Morgan, J. A. Hobson, and R. Stickgold
   2002. "Practice with sleep makes perfect: sleep-dependent motor skill learning." Neuron. Jul 3; 35(1):205–11.
Walters, A. S., R. J. Elin, B. Cohen, J. C. Moller, W. Oertel, and K. Stiasny-Kolster
   2007. "Magnesium not likely to play a major role in the pathogenesis of restless legs syndrome: serum and cerebrospinal fluid studies." Sleep Med. Mar; 8(2):186–7.
Wamsley, Erin J., and Robert Stickgold
   2011. "Memory, sleep and dreaming: experiencing consolidation." Sleep Med Clin. 6(1):97–108.
Waterhouse, J., G. Atkinson, B. Edwards, and T. Reilly
   2007. "The role of a short post-lunch nap in improving cognitive, motor, and sprint performance in participants with partial sleep deprivation." J Sports Sci. Dec; 25(14):1557–66.

Watson, N. F., et al

2015. "Recommended amount of sleep for a healthy adult: a joint consensus statement of the American Academy of Sleep Medicine and Sleep Research Society." J Clin Sleep Med. Jun 15; 11(6):591–2.

Weaver, Matthew

2015. "Greece crisis: what are the effects of sleep deprivation on decision-making?" *Guardian*. Jul 13.

Wehr, T. A.

1992. "In short photoperiods, human sleep is biphasic." J Sleep Res. 1(2):103–7.

Weinberg, Bennett Alan, and Bonnie Bealer

2002. *The Caffeine Advantage: How to Sharpen Your Mind, Improve Your Physical Performance, and Achieve Your Goals—the Healthy Way*. New York: Free Press.

Wilckens, K. A., S. G. Woo, A. R. Kirk, K. I. Erickson, and M. E. Wheeler

2014. "Role of sleep continuity and total sleep time in executive function across the adult lifespan." Psychol Aging. Sep; 29(3):658–65.

Wiley, T. S., and Bent Formby

2001. *Lights Out: Sleep, Sugar, and Survival*. New York: Atria Books.

Wilkinson, R. T., and K. B. Campbell

1984. "Effects of traffic noise on quality of sleep: assessment by EEG, subjective report, or performance the next day." J Acoust Soc Am. Feb; 75(2):468–75.

Williamson, A. M., and Anne-Marie Feyer

2000. "Moderate sleep deprivation produces impairments in cognitive and motor performance equivalent to legally prescribed levels of alcohol intoxication." Occup Environ Med. 57(10):649–55.

Wolfe, Tom

1975. *The Painted Word*. New York: Picador.

Wong, M. M., K. J. Brower, and R. A. Zucker

2009. "Childhood sleep problems, early onset of substance use and behavioral problems in adolescence." Sleep Med. 10(7):787–96.

Yoo, S. S., et al.

2007. "The human emotional brain without sleep—a prefrontal amygdala disconnect." Curr Biol. Oct 23; 17(20):R877–8.

Youngstedt, S. D.

2005. "Effects of exercise on sleep." Clin Sports Med. Apr; 24:355–65.

Zimecki, M.

2006. "The lunar cycle: effects on human and animal behavior and physiology." Postepy Hig Med Dosw. 60:1–7.

INDEX

(*continued*)

(continued)

(*continued*)

ABOUT THE AUTHORS

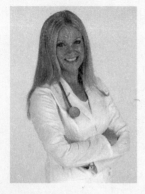

Terry Cralle, RN, MS, is cofounder of a four-bed sleep disorders center in Virginia and a nationally recognized sleep health consultant, educator, and advocate. Her work in the field of sleep medicine has ranged from patient care to clinical research and continuing education for nurses. As a certified clinical sleep educator, she is a highly sought-after consultant and speaker for schools, corporations, hospitals, and community organizations, as well as for the hospitality, travel, and bedding industry. Terry works closely with the International Sleep Products Association, Start School Later, and the Pajama Program. She is the national spokesperson for the Better Sleep Council. She is the author, with William David Brown, of *Snoozby and the Great Big Bedtime Battle*.

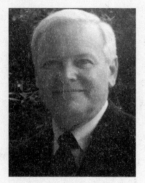

William David Brown, PhD, DABSM, CBSM (diplomate of the American Board of Sleep Medicine, certified in behavioral sleep medicine), has treated hundreds of patients for a full range of sleep disorders over the past two decades while serving as the clinical director of several sleep centers in Texas. A sleep psychologist at Children's Medical Center in Dallas, he is the primary clinician diagnosing and treating pediatric insomnia using behavioral techniques. Dr. Brown is also assistant professor of psychiatry at the University of Texas Southwestern Medical School in Dallas, where he obtained his training in sleep medicine. Dr. Brown is among an elite group of only two hundred doctors in the US who specialize in treating insomnia. He is also a fellow of the American Academy of Sleep Medicine. With Teofilo Lee-Chiong he is the author of *Focus on Sleep Medicine: A Self-Assessment* and editor of *Polysomnography, Volumes I and II*.

202-903-6066
Jose
202 873 787
ARCWE